Office Copy

SAY GOOD-BYE TO
ALLERGY-RELATED

AUTISM

By

Devi S. Nambudripad,

M.D., D.C., L.Ac., Ph.D.

Author of
Say Good-Bye to ... Series

This book has revolutionized
the Practice of Autism Treatment.

The doctor of the future will give no medicine,
But will interest his patients
In the care of the human frame, in diet,
And in the cause and prevention of disease.
                    -Thomas A. Edison

Published by
Delta Publishing Company
6714 Beach Blvd., Buena Park, CA 90621
(888) 890-0670, (714) 523-8900, Fax: (714) 523-3068
Web site: www.naet.com

Whole Body Wellness LLC

DEDICATION
This book is dedicated to
all Autistic Children and their Parents.

First Edition, 1999
Second Edition, 2006

Copyright © 2005 by Devi S. Nambudripad
M.D., D.C., L.Ac., Ph.D. (Acu.)
Buena Park, California
All rights reserved.

Library of Congress Control No: 2004105573

ISBN:0-9743915-6-5

Printed in U.S.A.

The medical information and procedures contained in this book are not intended as a substitute for consulting your physician. Any attempt to diagnose and treat an illness using the information in this book should come under the direction of an NAET physician who is familiar with this technique. Because there is always some risk involved in any medical treatment or procedure, the publisher and author are not responsible for any adverse effects or consequences resulting from the use of any of the suggestions or procedures in this book. Please do not use this book if you are unwilling to assume the risks. All matters regarding your health should be supervised by a qualified medical professional.

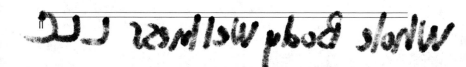

CONTENTS

Other Books by Dr. Nambudripad include:

Say Good-bye to Illness, 3rd Edition in English
Say Good-bye to Illness, 1st Edition in French
Say Good-bye to Illness, 1st Edition in Spanish
Say Good-bye to Illness, 1st Edition in German
Say Good-bye to Illness, 1st Edition in Japanese
Say Good-bye to Allergy-related Autism, 2nd. Edition
Say Good-bye to ADD and ADHD
Say Good-bye to Children's Allergies
Say Good-bye to Your Allergies
Say Good-bye to Asthma
Freedom From Environmental Sensitivities
Living Pain Free
The NAET Guide Book, 6th Edition

Books can also be ordered from www.naet.com

AUTISM TESTIMONIALS

NAET is truly awesome. You will want to pass this book on to others and spread the word about this amazing technique. Anyone who has wrestled with a rotation diet or tried to eliminate wheat, sugar and dairy from a small child's diet knows what a struggle that can be. But with the NAET process all of this becomes unnecessary. An allergen can be eliminated within 25 hours of treatment! No more having to avoid the food. By finding a NAET practitioner in your area, and following through with the treatments, you and your child can get a new lease on life and tackle new horizons.

Sandra C. Denton, MD
Alaska Alternative Medicine Clinic, LLC
3333 Denali St., Anchorage, AK 99503
(907) 563-6200

As a recently retired psychiatrist, I have witnessed the great devastation and feelings of helplessness, which many families have experienced by having an autistic child in the home. Now, with NAET, we finally have a treatment approach which is providing real improvement in these difficult cases. I applaud Dr. Devi for her great accomplishments in helping to relieve the suffering of her fellow humans.

Robert Prince, MD

NAET of North Carolina
Charlotte, NC
(704) 537-0201

NAET has changed my practice. NAET is a profound and fascinating technique of correcting allergy-related autism in children. In my experience of treating children using NAET since 1997, I have found the food and environmental allergies are the underlying causes of not only autism but most pediatric problems.

Sue Anderson, D.C.
Ann Arbor, MI
(734) 662-9140

My first autistic patient was a 29-year-old autistic adult. When he began treatment with me, he was unable to communicate with anyone about his needs. He was incontinent and was on diapers. He behaved like a two-year-old. When he finished the first five NAET basic treatments, he was able to communicate with his parents asking for his favorite food - ice cream. When he finished the mineral mix treatment, he stopped his bladder incontinence. By the time he completed his basic fifteen treatments, he was on his way to recovery. Step by step, little by little, I watched how NAET transformed a violent, frustrated, autistic adult into a passive, focused, manageable state. Ever since I have seen many autistic patients go through similar processes. When children get the NAET treatments at a young age the results are phenomenal. The younger the patients, the faster the results. NAET is a simple technique but it is powerful beyond imagination!

Mala Moosad, R.N., L.Ac., ND
Buena Park, CA
(714) 523-8900

I have been practicing NAET for 13 years. It has changed my practice greatly and has affected many lives positively including many autistic children I have treated over the years. Thank you Dr. Devi for helping me to make a difference in their lives!

Farangis Tavily, L.Ac.
20 Sunnyside Ave., A397
Mill Valley, CA 94941
(415) 302-7907

NAET Gave My Son Back!

My son was absolutely normal until 18 months old. He had begun speech and other normal activities for his age. He was left alone with other family members for one night since I had to go away to attend some family emergency. He cried the whole time I was gone and got high fever from crying. He also developed an ear infection. He was given antibiotics, repeatedly a few times. When he got better from his fever, he had lost the ability to speak and interact with others normally as before.

Finally he was diagnosed as having severe ADHD. I took him to many specialists all over the country. He remained nonverbal until 7 years old. Then I heard about Dr. Devi and read her book, "Say Good-bye to allergy-related Autism." My son had many allergies. Our whole family had numerous allergies. So I immediately called her office and traveled to Buena Park, CA. She began treating him right away. By the time he received 10 basic treatments, his allergic reactions were lessened. After about 25 treatments, he began speaking. As he got treated further, his communication and behavior, and other skills improved.

When he started with Dr. Devi, he had 38 prominent symptoms on the autism and allergy list. Now after treating for about 100 treatments in two year-period, he has four mild symptoms left behind. We have resolved 34 symptoms so far. I wish I had known about NAET sooner, then my son wouldn't have to remain nonverbal until 7 years old. I am home schooling him now. Parents, if you can take your child to NAET as soon as you can soon after you discover your child has autism or ADHD, recovery will be faster. If any parent would like to discuss NAET with me, please contact me at the address below. I will be glad to talk to you and give my testimonial.

"Roxie"
Phone: (480) 767-2728

These following testimonials are taken from "Amazon.com" book review section.

Steven, a seven year old autistic child began treatment on the same day when I started my treatment. I distinctly remember his appearance on the first day of his visit in Dr. Devi's office. He was bumping into things and people, had no awareness of the surroundings or people, was flapping his hands, pulling his sleeves, chewing his clothes, running back and forth in the waiting room aimlessly, etc. Then I didn't see him for a while, because we both had appointments at different times. I saw him the other day again, and I couldn't recognize him. His mother said he had 11 treatments. He has not yet treated for immunizations. He was sitting in the TV room with other children and watching TV calmly. What a transformation! I wonder why more people don't look for NAET or take their autistic children to NAET practitioners! Steven's dramatic changes forced me to read this book. What a book! Great information

Say Good-bye to Allergy-related Autism

for the parents of autistic children. As usual lots of useful self-help tips for the parents. This book is packed with information. Everyone with an autistic child or relative must read this book. This can give a new meaning to your life.

Karen, LA

This book, Say Good-bye to Allergy-Related Autism" is great! Especially helpful to us since we are currently treating our son via NAET. It does work and we have seen incredible, wonderful, changes in our son. After trying Western medicine, 7 doctors to be exact, to alternative methods such as P&N allergy treatments, we stumbled across NAET. This has saved us from many more years of heartache trying to help our son. It is noninvasive and we have never seen anything like it. I haven't met anyone yet who has actually done NAET with thier child who has said it hasn't worked for them. Do not listen to the nay sayers in here. From the lack of personal experience noted in the reviews it looks like they haven't even tried NAET, so how can they judge it? I just wish we would have found NAET before subjecting our son to all the doctors, the extensive blood work, the painful allergy tests, and ridiculous, next to impossible, special diets!!! Our son can actually have ice cream now at birthday parties at school. He's not in a special school, and through each treatment we are seeing more and more improvement in his speech! This book goes deeper into the mechanisms of how NAET can help the children that "Western" medicine has given up on and would rather medicate, and put into special schools, verses finding out the culprit behind their developmental issues! I highly recommend the book and NAET! This is the second time I have submitted this same review. My first review was never inserted for this book. For some reason Amazon.com would rather leave the negative, and unsubstantiated reviews online verses a first hand personal account of the true effects of this type of treatment. I hope for all parents sake and their precious children's sake, that this review will make it to thier screen so they can get on thier way to a life long recovery from this mystery illness. You don't have to do the special diets, undergo the tedious schooling, and medicate your child. NAET will show you how.

longlocks
(Texas)

ACKNOWLEDGMENTS

I am deeply grateful to my devoted husband, Kris K. Nambudripad, for his inspiration, encouragement and assistance in my schooling and later, in the formulation of this project. Without his cooperation in researching reference work, revision of manuscripts, word processing and proofreading, it is doubtful whether this book would ever have been completed. My sincere thanks also go to the many clients who have entrusted their care to me, for without them I would have had no case studies, no technique, and certainly no extensive source of personal research upon which to base this book.

I am also deeply grateful to the parents of Dominic, Steve, John, Steven, James, Matt, Brown, Mark, Ralph, Ann, Bob, Connie, Eric, Paul, Young, John, Sean, Maureen, Hrayr, and all other children whose names I haven't mentioned here due to lack of space, for believing in me from the very beginning of my research, supporting my theory and helping me conduct the on-going *detective* work. I want to express my special gratitude to Mary N. for showing such enthusiasm in not only taking care of her son's problem, but in sharing and spreading information about NAET to all autistic communities within her reach and constantly taking responsibility in educating other parents with similar problems. With the support of mothers (parents) like Mary, we will eliminate autism from the face of the earth soon.

I'd also like to thank Pras, Sara, Nath, Kart, Peyt and their parents for allowing me to take pictures and share with others to educate them about NAET. In addition I would like to express my heartfelt thanks to my friends who are excellent NAET practitioners and supported me by providing case studies, patients' testimonials, and constant encouragements to publish this second edition of this book. Without their ardent help, the writing of this book would have been only a dream.

Moreover, I wish to thank Mala and Mohan for allowing me to work on the book by relieving me from the daily clinical duties, and helping me in the formulation of this book. I do not have enough words to express my thanks to Robert Prince, M.D., Georgianne Allen and many of my friends who wish to remain anonymous for proofreading the work, and Mr. Roy M. at Delta Publishing for his printing expertise. I am deeply grateful for my professional training and the knowledge and skills acquired in classes and seminars on chiropractic and applied kinesiology at the Los Angeles College of Chiropractic in Whittier, California; the California Acupuncture College in Los Angeles; SAMRA University of Oriental Medicine, Los Angeles; University of Health Sciences, Antigua; and the clinical experience obtained at the clinics attached to these colleges.

My special thanks also go to the late Dr. Richard F. Farquhar at Farquhar Clinic, where I accumulated many hours of special instruction in kinesiology which led me to improve the NAET.

I extend my sincere thanks to my great teachers. They have helped me to grow immensely at all levels. My professional mentors are also indirectly responsible for the improvement of my personal health, as well as, that of my family, patients and other NAET practitioners among whom also are included countless doctors of Western and Oriental medicine, chiropractic, osteopathy, allopathy, in addition to their patients.

Many of the nutritionists instrumental in this process of developing NAET were professors at the institutions previously mentioned. Their willingness and complete dedication to teaching, coupled with their commitment of personal time to give the interviews necessary to complete this work, places them beyond my mere expressions of gratitude. They are living testaments to the greatest ideals of the medical profession.

Devi S. Nambudripad,
M.D., D.C., L..Ac., Ph.D. (Acu.)
Los Angeles, CA

Say Good-bye to Allergy-related Autism

PREFACE

For years, autism was considered a type of mild brain disorder with no known cure. Even now, not many people know that autism is reversible. So many intricate messages and signals are necessary for us to receive, process, and retrieve information that one miscue, or blockage to the brain might hinder us from communicating normally with another person.

For years, any abnormality of the brain was considered a type of madness. Autism was included in that category by lay people. People were frightened of persons with any brain disorders even if it happened to their close family members. Most of the people with brain disorders ended up being labeled as having mental illness (madness) in those days. The mentally sick people were treated badly by their family and friends or were committed to mental institutions. Historically some believed mental illness was a hereditary disorder while other people believed mental illness was due to a person being possessed by devils or evil spirits.

Such assumptions and fears produced various exotic treatments like exorcism, (trying to remove the possessed entities by inflicting pain on the sufferer, burning body parts of the sufferer, etc.), warding off evil spirits by chanting positive affirmation, or reciting certain religious words, chanting religious songs, etc. Many people were afraid to be associated with a family who had a mentally ill person in it. Other families in town avoided them and would not get involved in relationships with them, especially marriage. People were afraid that they might become "crazy" by fraternizing with them, thus creating fear and isolation in the family members of the victim.

So the family of the "crazy" person did not want anyone else to find out the truth about their sick family member. Therefore, in order to seem like a normal family, many chose to hide the person from the community. They locked him/her up in a secluded room, perhaps in a dungeon, basement, or in a soundproof room in the house, hidden from the rest of the world.

As I was growing up in a rural village in India, I knew of a few innocent people who became victims of such ignorance and spent their lives in total seclusion until they died. The causes of their mental illness were never found. No one other than some immediate family members, or immediate neighbors knew of their existence. One such case was an autistic adult. At that time, I did not know she was autistic. Now, after learning more about autism, and examining and treating patients who suffer from different stages of autism, I know she was just autistic, but labeled as mentally sick.

This disorder was probably prevalent in villages and towns all over the world. Autism is not a new age health disorder. It was prevalent all over the world years ago. Few people talked about it or tried to cure the affected person. They were kept isolated, labeled as mentally unstable, or mentally retarded, while only a few people tried to help them overcome their illnesses; however, almost no one knew how to help these people.

One of the families I knew in my childhood was sad to have two of their offsprings born mentally retarded (None of these people had received any type of childhood immunizations or vaccinations, because there were none available in the place where I grew up in those days). They used to bring doctors from different fields to help their children. One type of treatment given to them interested me, so I watched the procedure many times. These teenage patients were made to lie flat on their backs (if they did not cooperate, they were restrained), their heads were kept soaked in a herbal concoction with cold pressed sesame oil for a few hours daily, for 41 days at a time, in order to cool their "hot" brain and nervous system. Those herbal doctors thought the mental instability was due to excess heat in the brain.

Chinese medicine also holds similar principles regarding mental instabilies. It teaches that liver fire can rise to the brain and cause heat in the brain, thus resulting in mental derangement. The dampness from gall bladder, phlegm from the spleen and cold mist from the heart (due to blockages in respective meridians) reach the brain and cause from poor to no mental clarity and severe mental instability. Chinese diagnosis makes better sense since we find the gallbladder, spleen, heart and kidney meridians are the ones usually affected in autistic children.

Today we know that many mental disorders are due to various nutritional deficiencies, or chemical imbalances of the brain brought on by nutritional deficiencies. In most cases, these deficiencies may not be due to failing to consume nutritious food, but may be due to allergies to nutritional elements in food. These allergies cause poor digestion, absorption and assimilation of the essential nutrients, which are the precursors to various brain enzymes.

In the absence of essential nutrients, brain enzymes and neurotransmitters are not formulated normally. However, taking enzyme supplements without removing the allergy to them is not the answer. If the person is not allergic to the enzymes, appropriate enzyme supplementation will help. But if the person is allergic to the enzyme supplements, he/she can get worse. These incomplete brain enzymes can cause malfunctions of various parts of the brain and nervous system leading to abnormal behaviors, including autism, attention deficit hyperactive disorders, schizophrenia, bipolar disorders, manic depressive disorders, anxiety disorders, and various kinds of depression.

Many parents today, just as in the past, prefer to keep the brain-related health disorders of their children as secretive as possible. Unfortunately, autism is one of them. Over the years, I have treated numerous cases of autistic children and adults, suffering from varying degrees of autism, with good success. When the children get well, some parents become reluctant to share their improvement or journey from autism to normalcy with others. They are happy that their children got well but not willing to be reminded of their past nightmare. They don't want their children to know their troubled past either. They don't want anyone to know that their child had autism.

One mother of my patient, a native of another country, said that no one in her family (except her husband) knew that her daughter had autism. She brought her to the U.S and

Europe for treatments. If her relatives knew that her child was autistic, it would damage the child's future since autism in her country is still looked upon as insanity. She would have difficulty putting her in a regular school, and later finding a husband for her. Even though she gave her testimonials, I had to promise her that I would never ever reveal her real name, under any circumstances.

This is not only happening to foreign born parents, this is also happening in the United States. I have a few autistic children as patients, whose parents are well known doctors, lawyers, investors and actors, who refuse to give their identity or give permission to have their names associated with autism. The fear of their future image is the concern here.

When I realized that most autistic disorders I treated were allergy-based, my passion to inform and educate people grew. In the meantime, many of my patients and my friends insisted that I put this valuable information in a book form, since the best form of education is through published materials. Consequently, "Say Good-bye to Allergy-related Autism," came into being.

Fortunately, I have a few fearless, compassionate, caring parents who are excited with the possibilities that not only their children, but also all other autistic children of the world could have a chance to start over, and have a new hopeful life, with NAET. They are willing to go all the way to educate other parents of autistic children, provide support, and share information about NAET. With the help of these committed and caring parents, we hope to achieve our dream—to reach all the autistic communities of the world and make NAET available to all in need of treatment. We applaud and extend our heartfelt thanks to these selfless, caring, humanitarian parents who are eager to see world autism brought under control.

We have a lot of work ahead for us if we want people to accept autism as a treatable deficiency disease, rather than an incurable mental disorder. If we want autism to be accepted as one of the health disorders caused by allergies, we need to educate the parents, children, and the public about autism.

We just completed a clinical trial, a pilot study with 60 children of both sexes, ages ranging between 3 and 10 years, 30 children in the treatment group and 30 in the control group. Halfway evaluation report looked very promising. The final report will not be ready for a couple of months since it takes time to collect all the reports from the laboratories and various assessing departments. From a practical perspective, we have over 20 out of 30 (66%) have moved to regular school activities according to the reports we received from the children's school. The exact percentage will be released only after receiving the final reports. We hope (including our staff, volunteers, and the parents) this pilot study result will help the skeptics and nonbelievers to understand and provide their support in bringing unfortunate children with autism out of their shells.

We know now that an autistic child has deficiencies in seeing, hearing, and perceiving things as a normal child would. We also know that most of these functional deficiencies are in fact due to allergies at least with children with allergy-based autism. These children are born with allergic tendencies, suffer from various allergy-related health problems since birth and they could become allergic to anything like food, drinks, food additives, food colors, chemicals. environmental toxins, heavy metal toxins, other external toxins, drug-induced allergies, defective DNA, defective brain parts, etc.

In this book, technical terms are kept to a minimum. Although I do use some specialized terminology, which may give some lay readers a harder time and diminish their reading pleasure and understanding, a glossary has been included. Caution has also been exercised in determining the depth of the subject matter; for instance, the way allergies and the nervous system are inextricably interrelated, is just now being understood. But since the human nervous system is one of the most complex areas of human anatomy and remains largely uncharted, I decided to deal with it in a sweeping fashion, drawing the reader's attention only to the close link between the nervous system and allergic reactions.

After learning about the prevalence of allergies in children with autism and gathering a great deal of clinical hands-on experience with my young patients from my 22 years of practice as an allergist, I felt motivated to write this book on allergy-based Autism and how to conquer it with NAET. I would feel gratified, indeed, if the up-to-date material compiled in this book were to contribute to the well-being of a great number of Autistic children, and give their worried and frustrated parents peace of mind.

My dream then would be fulfilled, if this book could provide help to the tired, frustrated mothers of Autistic children, in managing their symptoms efficiently or reducing their symptoms or completely eliminating their symptoms and help them to become productive people. If NAET could reach the misdiagnosed and wrongly treated Autistic children in the community, help the children whether they are truly autistic or suffering from autistm-like symptoms, help the children to become calm, responsible and productive individuals, I would then feel that my job is done.

NAET combines various healing elements from different disciplines of medicine, including allopathy (traditional Western medicine), acupuncture and acupressure, chiropractic, kinesiology, and nutrition. It is a non-invasive, drug-free holistic treatment. There is a strong emphasis on Traditional Chinese Medicine (TCM), including acupuncture or acupressure. Because of this, you might want to familiarize yourself with acupuncture/acupressure techniques. An in-depth introduction to Oriental medicine was neither intended nor considered appropriate within the scope of this publication.

To enhance your understanding of the subject matter contained herein, you might check some of the other relevant books and articles quoted as a part of this book. You will also find numerous sources in the Bibliography.

Welcome! Say good-bye to allergy-related autism!

Dr. Devi S. Nambudripad,
M.D., D.C., L.Ac., Ph.D. (Acu.)
Los Angeles, California

INTRODUCTION

I t is your child's human right to grow up in a normal environment and live a normal life by eating whatever he/she wants, wearing normal clothes, attending regular school, and playing like other children. You are with your child most of the time. No one understands your child as you do. If your child is unable to do any of these things, you need to attend to the matter immediately. If any abnormalities are noted you should have your child checked immediately. If there is any problem detected, you should get professional help right away. The sooner you look into the problem, the better the prognosis or outcome.

When I look back into my childhood days, I recall the multitude of health problems I suffered. I now know that they may have followed an allergy to whatever I ate, touched or inhaled. I literally lived on prescription medicines and herbs to control my symptoms. No one knew how to find the cause of my heath problems. No one knew how to test the allergy using neuromuscular sensitivity testing (also known as muscle response testing) in those days. In fact the word "allergy" was nonexistent in the part of the world where I grew up. People got sick there, but no one had any allergies. As an infant, I had severe infantile eczema, which lasted until I was seven or eight-years-old. I was given Western medicine and Ayurvedic herbal medicine without a break. When I was eight-years-old, one of the herbal doctors told my parents to feed me white rice cooked with a special herb formula. This special diet helped me a great deal. The herbalist seemed to know what he was doing. But it didn't cure my problem. It only gave temporary relief until I discovered NAET.

In 1976, I relocated to Los Angeles. I became more health-conscious and tried to eat healthy by adding more whole grain products and complex carbohydrates into my daily bland diet. All of a sudden, I became very ill. I suffered from repeated bronchitis, pneumonia and my arthritis returned. My symptoms multiplied, I suffered from insomnia, clinical depression, constant sinusitis and frequent migraine headaches. I felt extremely tired all the time, but I remained wide-awake when I went to bed. I tried many different antibiotics and medicines, changed doctors, and consulted nutritionists. All the medications, vitamins and herbs made me sicker, and the consumption of good nutrition made me worse. I was nauseated all the time, every inch of my body ached; I lived on aspirin and water to keep me going.

I searched everywhere for an answer to my agony. Through my illness and devastation, I continued my search. Whenever I signed up for a class in some health subject that I have never heard of before, or joined a new school to explore more on health, my husband used to make a statement "You are a glutton for punishment" and I would reply, "This glutton is going to be off the punishment soon." I longed to be free of pain at least for a few days but I didn't know how.

While I was a student of Oriental medicine and attending one of the courses in electromagnetic energy and its interference with the human body and other surrounding objects, I arrived at a discovery, which resulted in the foundation of my own good health and that of my family. The integration of the relevant techniques from the various fields I studied, combined with my own discoveries, has since become the focus of my life to help my family, myself, and my patients. We were an allergic family — father-mother-son! We were allergic to almost everything around us. There was no known successful method of treatment for food allergies then (actually not even now in the year of 2005, as I am writing this), using Western medicine except avoidance, which means deprivation and frustration. Each of the disciplines I studied provided bits of knowledge, which I used to develop this new allergy elimination treatment now called Nambudripad's Allergy Elimination Techniques or NAET for short.

The more extensively I studied the subject of allergies, the more I found it to be a truly fascinating, yet highly complex field. Although food allergies as causes for multiple physiological problems, have been gaining acceptance as a separate area of medical study in the last few years, it certainly has not been given the recognition it deserves. In fact, knowledge of the field is still quite limited not only among the general public, but also among those who treat allergies, because of the limited volume of research conducted.

I can relate to the plight of parents searching for a cure for their children's illness, running from Western medical doctors to alternative forms of medicine, hoping for some assurance that their child will be able to lead a normal life. After exhausting their energy and finances, most parents face a grim future without getting much help. If your child's autism is allergy related, unless you eliminate the allergies, your child may not be able to function normally even if you feed him/her any amount of expensive, good nutrition. You need to find your child's allergies. Now there is an easy way to do that. You have to learn the testing techniques if you want to see your child functioning normally. I would like to see all parents learn and master this simple testing technique. Please read Chapter Six and practice to perfection. Then you will know how to help your child.

This book *Say Good-bye to Allergy-Related Autism* will guide you in searching for any possible abnormalities in your child, and assist you in finding the right help for your child. This book reveals the secrets of a remarkable breakthrough in medical history. This new treatment, NAET (Nambudripad's Allergy Elimination Techniques), approaches health care from a new intelligent viewpoint.

Say Good-bye to Allergy-Related Autism is filled with so much common sense, that it simply cannot be ignored by anyone who wants to lead a normal life. In an allergic person the brain and central nervous system react to foods (egg white, milk casein, milk albumin, wheat products, gluten, candida, refined starches, fatty acids, minerals, amino acids, turkey and serotonin, chocolate), heavy metals, chemicals, vaccines, immunizations and other substances as if they were poison, when they are really neutral, or in some cases beneficial. You can now reprogram your brain or your child's brain for perfect health by eliminating and/or neutralizing the adverse effects and side effects of allergens, and improve or restore the brain function.

Chiropractic, acupuncture and kinesiology techniques have already been proven and accepted in the medical world. It is important to note that these procedures along with my discovery of NAET will be beneficial to children suffering from Autism, ADHD (Attention Deficit Hyperactivity Disorder), and other learning disabilities.

If the autistic children are allowed to remain without treatment, they are unable to attend regular school, unable to find jobs, unable to live by themselves, and they become dependent on others for the rest of their lives. On the contrary, if they get treated for their allergies, and obtain proper schooling, they may be able to function in a normal fashion. They may be able to find jobs and live on their own with minimal help from others. Mild cases of autism and PDD can have complete reversal provided they receive appropriate treatment from an early age or as soon as problems are discovered. So it is for everyone's benefit to begin NAET treatments as early as possible.

WHAT IS AUTISM?

Autism is a nutritional deficiency disorder causing biological, neurological and developmental problems in children. The nutritional deficiency is not caused by failing to take enough nutrients by mouth but by poor digestion, absorption, assimilation and utilization of essential nutrients due to allergies. Autistic children are not digesting whatever they consume and their bodies do not receive essential nutrients from food or supplements they take.

Normal body functions cannot take place when there is insufficient amount of nutrients available in the body. Adequate amounts of nutrients are necessary for normal growth, development as well as for various enzymatic functions. Body functions will take place regularly with or without proper nutrients. In an allergic person when the appropriate nutrients are not assimilated or utilized adequately, the body will begin to substitute with other available substances to run the regular functions. The substituted substances will produce various health disorders and abnormal body functions as seen in autistic children.

Usually autistic children are born normal unless they are born with some genetic defects. Children are born with enough nutrients in their bodies which last for a while. By the time the storages run out, they are supposed to absorb and assimilate more nutrients from breast milk and other foods they consume on a daily basis. But if they are allergic to them they do not get any from the food they eat. Eventually, the food storage gets empty and substitution of nutrients begins to conduct the routine body functions. Soon they begin to develop functional abnormalities. Before the age of three usually their symptoms become more noticeable.

According to various studies, it has been found that the growth and development of the brain takes place before the age of five.

Growth and development of the brain need appropriate nutrients. When the allergic children lack nutrients, their brains do not develop properly. When they do not digest, absorb or assimilate fats, insulation of nerve cells with myelin does not take place properly. This makes them abnormally sensitive to different stimuli causing them to have abnormal body movements (like twisting, hand flapping, hair pulling, etc.), disturbances in the rate of appearance of physical, social and language skills and severe impairment in communication and social interactions. Toxins from the allergens cause accumulation of water in the body and brain causing the person not to hear properly, not to see properly, not to comprehend or recognize the sounds the child hears due to poor differentiation of the voices or sounds due to water retention. Imagine you are sitting on the floor of a swimming pool trying to listen to someone's talk from outside the pool. You may hear some sounds but may not able to hear them clearly. We can understand the condition when one gets an attack of common cold. In some instances, we experience severe congestion above neck making the head feel heavy and numb. While going through the initial stages of a common cold, we could suffer from cerebral allergy and we may feel that our brains are swollen making the hearing function diminished. An allergy is the major cause of common cold. When the allergy affects different tissues of the brain we experience the symptoms of the energy blockages of the particular tissue. In the autistic individual, each and every allergen he/she comes in contact directly targets the brain causing him/her to have the feeling of "cold" all the time. So their vision is impaired, hearing is impaired and speech is impaired until he/she avoids all the allergens or get treated through NAET. The protective function of the blood-brain barrier may not be functional either. When they get exposed to strong allergens (heavy metal poisoning, antibiotics and immunization drugs to which they are allergic, carbon monoxide, pesticides, bacterial toxins, viral toxins, strong chemicals like carpet cleaning liquids), their brains get affected immediately leading to various brain-related symptoms: like autism, ADD, ADHD, learning disability, dyslexia, depression, anger, behavioral disturbances, etc. Any of these allergens can act as a trigger to the child who has a strong inheritance for allergies (having parents or grandparents with food or environmental sensitivities and suffering from Asthma, eczema, migraines, arthritis, etc.). We have also noticed that most mothers of autistic children suffered from gestational diabetes and/or yeast infections during pregnancy. These children probably may have been already suffering from various allergies from birth (colicky pains, constipation, abdominal distention, asthma, eczema, insomnia, frequent crying). This child may also have the brain as the weakest organ in his/her body causing the brain to become the target organ for any allergic reaction. In such children any of these allergens can act as a trigger to bring out autism-like reactions to the surface.

The brain and the network of the nervous system do not function normally in autistic people. It seems that the cranial nerves become swollen causing inability to see, smell, and hear, think or talk normally. Their vision becomes foggy, and images get scrambled causing unclear pictures to float in front of them, because of blockages in the nerves supplying the vision center. That's the reason autistic children do not look at you or look into your eyes when you talk to them. They cannot smell, because the cranial nerve that is responsible for smell is not getting an adequate nerve energy supply. They cannot hear normally due to poor nerve energy supply to the acoustic nerves. Their thinking, creativity, and imagination are minimal or muddled, because the nerves and brain tissue that are responsible for such functioning are not able to do their jobs due to the poor energy supply. Autistic people cannot speak because their speech center is not receiving messages from other areas to initiate speech or voice. Their sense of fine touch is also impaired. Something in their bodies, cause swelling of the tissue, especially in the brain and cranial nerves; thus disturbing the energy supply to the different parts of the brain that are responsible for the functioning of the five senses. From my experience in treating autistic children and adults, I have found that the cranial nerves are highly affected, making the midbrain area most affected in autistic people.

Autism is on the rise. According to 2005 statistics released from Center for Disease Control, one out of 166 children in cities and one out of 500 in other areas are being diagnosed as autistic in U.S. If the statistics is correct about the rate of increase of autism, then the situation is dreadful.

WHAT IS NAET?

NAET (Nambudripad's Allergy Elimination techniques) was discovered in 1983. NAET is a blend of medical knowledge and procedures compiled from all existing medical disciplines. NAET is able to eliminate allergies permanently without any future appearances of adverse reactions from the treated allergens. When the allergies are gone allergy sufferers can resume normal lives. That's how NAET can help with autism.

We study, read and see many health disorders around us every day. We recognize or diagnose them from their history, presenting symptoms and the laboratory tests supporting the symptoms. We prescribe, give and take various herbs, prescription and nonprescription medications to get the symptoms under control. When the pain and/or discomfort gets better we are happy and we don't bother to look into the cause that initiated the symptoms. Then the next episode occurs. The same routine is repeated. When the symptoms are gone, few people have the time or interest to look into the cause. Here is an example:

"I was sick yesterday and I couldn't go to school," Jane said.

Maria asked, "What was your problem?"

"I had a headache," Jane replied.

Jane's headache becomes the cause and the sickness. So the symptom becomes the cause to most people. People all over the world are looking at symptoms and treating symptoms. Instead, one should look for causes, as well as treat the symptoms.

It is different in NAET. Whatever the symptoms may be, we look for the cause. If we can trace the cause, NAET works faster. If a patient comes to my office with a headache, I will ask, "What caused your headache?" If the patient doesn't have a clue, NAET has a way to find the cause of the presenting symptoms.

All certified NAET practitioners know how to find causes. They may be the pear you ate at lunch; or the makeup you put on your face during your lunch break, or the perfume you smelled from one of your customers, or the candy bar you ate from the vending machine while returning from lunch; any of these could have triggered this headache. A NAET practitioner will probe until he/she finds the culprit. When you treat the allergy towards the offending substance the pain and discomfort will clear swiftly, never to return again in most cases.

NAET treatments for autism are more effective when patients are very young. The older they get, the longer it takes to treat successfully. I have treated autistic patients who were in their late twenties or early thirties, one of whom was 29 years old, I will call him Jack.

No one suspected Jack's problem stemmed from allergy. He was tall, weighed about 170 pounds, was well-built physically, and he was very strong, but had the mind of a three-year-old. When he had a successful treatment, one could tell he felt better by the way he would grab his short, slim father in such a tight embrace that it hurt. Other times, he jumped around in the hallway, like a little boy. Whenever he lost a treatment he grew very agitated, angry, physically violent towards his parents and caretakers, bit his own hand until it hurt him, and other times he banged his head against the concrete floor or the brick wall. His behaviors were so violent, my other patients and staff were afraid to be near him. I had to schedule him during our days off, and had to suggest that his father medicate him, to calm him down during the NAET treatment. If the symptoms are kept under control, NAET works better.

When children are small, someone can hold them and control them from physical violence to themselves or others; but when autistic children grow up without treatments, it may not be easy to manage them in a regular clinic. If they have violent and aggressive behaviors, they should be treated with NAET in special clinics or in a hospital, where more help is available. Calming medication or herbs should be given, after checking and clearing the allergy for the drug or herb. It is better to give a non-allergic drug or herb and keep them calm, rather than let them become violent and agitated during the NAET treatment, and during the 25 hours waiting period. Physical strength, of unmanaged autistic adults, is usually very high and you may need more people to help with the treatment. It may be exhausting for the patient, doctor, and the assistants. The treatments may not proceed smoothly if their nerves remain agitated.

There are many special schools and clinics in the U.S today where the autistic children are taught various behavior modifications. Specially trained people are available there to help bring your child to the wide world as a normal human being. If NAET is provided along with behavior modification, your child will grow to be a healthy, happy normal adult.

More than 8,000 patients with a variety of health problems have been treated with NAET and have achieved very satisfactory results in my office alone. From my own health improvements and watching and hearing about the thousands who have achieved similar results from my patients as well as from patients of other NAET practitioners, I am convinced that most of the ailments we see around us stem from allergies, including Autism.

WHAT IS AN ALLERGY?

A condition of unusual sensitivity of an individual, to one or more substances; which may be inhaled, swallowed, or contacted by the skin. These substances may be harmless or even beneficial, to the majority of other individuals. In sensitive individuals, contact with these substances (allergens) can produce a variety of symptoms in varying degrees, ranging from slight ADHD to Autism, mild itching to swelling of the tissues and organs, mild runny nose to severe asthmatic attacks, general tiredness to extreme fatigue, or life threatening anaphylaxis.

The ingested, inhaled, injected or contacted allergen is capable of alerting the immune system of the body. The frightened and confused immune system then commands the white blood cells to produce immunoglobulins to stimulate the release of neuro-chemical defense forces like histamines from the mast cells. These chemical mediators are released as part of the body's immune response.

If you carefully evaluate any health disorders, you may find an allergic factor involved in almost everything, including physical, physiological, psychological, and genetic disorders; likewise, autism is not any different.

Let us look at some examples:

A fourteen-year-old boy hurt his knees, sprained his ankles many times within a year while playing soccer. He was found to be allergic to his shin splints, cotton socks and shoes. After he was successfully treated for the above items with NAET, he was able to play soccer and take part in normal sports activities without a problem for the rest of his school years.

Say Good-bye to Allergy-related Autism

A 36-year-old man hurt his lower back while playing tennis. He had to be carried into the doctor's office in excruciating pain. He was found to be allergic to the fish meal he had before playing tennis. After he was treated for the abalone fish, he was able to walk out of the office in 30 minutes and play tennis the next day.

A 37-year-old female suffered from high blood pressure (190/120 mm of hg.) for six months. She was found to be allergic to the new mattress she had bought six months earlier. When she was successfully treated for the mattress, her blood pressure became normal.

A 43-year-old female, who was diagnosed as having schizophrenic disorders, was found to be allergic to many food groups in her daily diet. She was also allergic to household cleaning chemicals, soaps, detergents and pets. She was successfully treated for all of the above and became a normal productive individual again. She returned to school, completed her education, found a job that pays her a large sum, went off of permanent disability on her own, and now leads a normal, productive life.

A 28-year-old man suffered from extreme depression in the early morning hours. He lived by the ocean in Southern California. He was allergic to the morning cold air and fog. When he was treated for cold air mixed with cold mist, his years-long depression disappeared.

A 14-year-old boy with severe backache, joint pains and bone and muscle aches was found to be allergic to every food group he ate and everything he drank, including water. His paternal grandfather suffered a crippling kind of arthritis from a very young age. His father also suffered from severe joint pains and muscle aches, which did not respond to analgesics. He was told by previous medical practitioners who examined him that his health problems were genetic in origin. Nothing could be done except to learn to live with the pain. When he was treated for all his food allergies, he became free from his incurable pain.

A 65-year-old male suffered from frequent memory lapses and seizures that resembled some form of epilepsy, Alzheimer's disease or perhaps a mild stroke. He would often wander off in total confusion or complete amnesia, sometimes losing track of significant blocks of time. Neurological examination and a CAT scan showed his brain wave pattern to be completely normal. After considerable detective work, the cause in this case turned out to be the airborne spores of a fern tree he had recently planted in his backyard. He became absolutely normal after he was treated successfully for the same fern tree.

WHAT CAUSES ALLERGIES?

• Heredity - inherited from parents, grandparents, ancestors, etc.

• Toxins - produced in the body from: food interactions, unsuitable proteins, bacterial or viral infections, molds, yeast, fungus or parasitic infestation, vaccinations and immunizations, drug reactions, or constant contact with certain irritants like mercury, lead, copper, and various chemicals

• Low immune system function - due to surgeries, chronic illnesses, injury, long term starvation, etc.

• Radiation - excessive exposure to television, sun, radioactive materials, etc.

• Emotional factors

WHAT ARE SOME COMMON ALLERGENS?

• Inhalants: pollens, flowers, perfume, dust, paint, formaldehyde, etc.

• Ingestants: food, drinks, vitamins, drugs, food additives, etc.

• Contactants: fabrics, chemicals, cosmetics, furniture, utensils, etc.

• Injectants: insect bites, stings, injected drugs, vaccines, immunization, etc.

• Infectants: viruses, bacteria, contact with infected persons, etc.

• Physical Agents: heat, cold, humidity, dampness, fog, wind, dryness, sunlight, sound, etc.

• Genetic Factors: inherited illnesses or tendency from parents, grandparents, etc.

• Molds and Fungi: molds, yeast, candida, parasites, etc.

• Emotional Factors: painful memories of various incidents from past and present.

HOW DO I KNOW IF MY CHILD HAS ALLERGIES?

If you notice any unusual or strange behavior for the age of your child, that may give you the first clue. If he/she experiences any allergic symptoms or unusual physical, physiological or emotional symptoms in the presence of any of the above listed allergens, you can suspect an allergy contributing towards such changes.

WHO SHOULD USE THIS BOOK?

All parents, teachers, medical professionals, and anyone involved with a child with learning disorders should read this book; both to learn about NAET and to include NAET with your current mode of treatment as a way to enhance the results of your current treatment. This drug-free, non-invasive technique is ideal to treat infants, children, and grown-ups alike, as a means of removing the adverse reactions to allergens.

HOW IS THIS BOOK ORGANIZED?

When autism is reversed the real angel hiding within your child will get a chance to come out of the cage of autism. The front cover of the book demonstrates the results of NAET. The cover design is by one of our children who was once treated for ADHD, and who is now a smart, productive young man.

Chapter 1 - Autism is Treatable - explains the definition of allergy in various disciplines of medicine and also in laymen's terms and how it affects an autistic child. There are numerous autism case studies throughout the book, some are from the author's observation, some are from other NAET practitioners' case notes, and some are from the parents of children who have benefited from NAET.

Chapter 2 - Categories of Allergens - describes the various categories of allergens and how they can mimic autism.

Chapter 3 - Autism Screening Modalities - explains Autism Screening methods and Nambudripad's Testing Procedures (NTP).

This chapter gives you information about various allergy testing techniques.

Chapter 4 - Is it truly Autism? - is a step-by-step method of evaluating your child's allergic history.

Chapter 5 - The missing Link. - describes the normal function of the human nervous system and how it creates allergies by receiving wrong stimuli.

Chapter 6 - NAET Testing Procedures - discusses kinesiology, acupuncture and how energy blockages can cause allergies and diseases in the human body. It also explains Neuromuscular Sensitivity Testing (NST) to detect allergies, the main testing technique used in NAET testing procedures.

Chapter 7 - Symptoms of the Meridians - explains the pathological functions of major acupuncture meridians.

Chapter 8 - Helping your Child - describes and illustrates self-balancing techniques and the use of acupressure techniques to give the reader more control over his/her child's reactions. It describes various self-help modalities to balance your child's brain and nervous system with illustrations for better understanding of the procedure.

Chapter 9 - NAET Allergens - explains the basic NAET allergens, the most effective treatment approach and the order of treatments.

Chapter 10- Autism Case Studies - various case studies are offered here in detail including the procedure, the immediate reactions, the immediate response and reactions, and responses after leaving the office during 25 hours after treatment

Actual parents' testimonials are also included where appropriate, to help the reader understand the severity of the symptoms, the process involved in undergoing treatment, and to eliminate allergic reactions in order to reverse autism. This is done for two purposes:

1. To provide guidance to an inexperienced NAET practitioner in treating autism successfully.

2. To provide an understanding of NAET to the parents and the type of reactions and responses they could expect for their child after each treatment.

Chapter 11- Nutrition Corner - emphasizes the importance of essential nutritional elements in your child's diet.

Chapter 12 - Eliminate Autism through NAET- describes author's dream to eliminate this devastating disorder - autism from the world, permanently. Is it possible? Yes, absolutely, if we all work together it is possible.

The Glossary will help you to understand the appropriate meanings of the medical terminology used in certain parts of the book.

The Resource Guide is provided to assist you in finding products and consultants to support you in dealing with allergies and autism.

The Bibliography covers numerous sources of information on autism.

A detailed Index is included to help you locate your area of interest quickly and easily.

ABBREVIATIONS USED IN THIS BOOK:

EAV: Electro Acupuncture by Voll

NAET: Nambudripad's Allergy Elimination Techniques

NARF: Nambudripad's Allergy Research Foundation

NTP: Nambudripad's Testing Procedures

NST: Neuromuscular Sensitivity Testing

MRT: Muscle Response Testing

1

AUTISM IS TREATABLE

I t was 3:00 A.M. and my two-year-old son, Dominic, was humming along to the song, "A Whole New World.." It had been another rough night for him as he had awakened at 1:00 A.M. screaming and banging his head. He had finally settled down after an hour, and had requested the Aladdin video as usual. As he drifted off to sleep, I sat there watching him. He seemed so peaceful now. It was hard to believe, when he had settled down, that he was the same little boy.

I began to wonder, as I had so many times before, what made it so hard for my little one to live in our world? What happened to the little baby who used to smile at me? Where had he gone? What "new world" had he entered? I said a prayer for him, and then I prayed for strength and for an answer that would bring our son back to us.

Dominic had cried more than average since the day he was born; the doctors had told me it was colic and sent me on my way. Even so, he had been a happy baby, eager to play and be cuddled. Yet, by 15- months-old, he became belligerent with his crying episodes. He would often bang his head and throw himself on the ground in a rage. There was no consoling him, as he resisted all comforting, although he did allow only me to try.

The doctors did not have an explanation for me and so my husband and I just sat there night after night trying to help our son as he would cling to us, and then push us away. At one point, I called 911 because I thought he was having a seizure. He also had other physical problems such as diarrhea, rashes, hives, stuffy nose, runny nose, fluid in the ears, and earaches. Dominic's sleep was often interrupted by these attacks. At 18 months he began to appear withdrawn from the world around him. When he would visit relatives he would hide in a corner or under my chair. The pediatrician thought it was the "terrible two's" stage that was responsible for his tantrums and strange behavior. Yet, in my heart, I knew differently. My husband and I were exhausted, and I felt so alone.

Then one day, a special friend of mine handed me Dr. Devi's book, *Say Good-bye to Illness.* Until then, I had not heard of alternative therapies, like acupuncture, acupressure, or chiropractic. I was completely dependent on Western medicine and Western medical doctors. I did not have much time, and never thought of going to bookstores to look for health alternatives, because I thought only Western medicine exists to cure us from our health problems. I was simply not educated by anyone about any alternative medical therapies. I wish there had been, and would be more exposure and discussion about alternative medical therapies and their benefits and importance in our daily lives. There may be millions of desperate mothers all over the world, thinking that they have to use just Western medical therapies to get well. Many of them may be suffering due to mere ignorance.

Well, I had tried Western medicine all along and I had failed to see any results. So I decided to take him to Dr. Devi. Dominic was 100% allergic to 156 items. We began treatments and Dominic began to get some relief. During the initial treatment days, when he would have an attack, we would massage his acupressure points that Dr. Devi taught us to use, and he would relax into my arms. My husband would have to hold him down as I massaged his points, because he was very strong during his attacks. At this point, Dominic hardly spoke a word. He would speak in jargon and no one could understand him. He would easily become overwhelmed, and was resistant to any change in his routines. Dominic would run in circles and flap his arms. He would hold food in his mouth for an hour at a time, and would nervously chew holes in his shirt.

He was tested by a regional center, and was found to be a year and a half behind in his language and fine motor skills.

He was then referred to a specialist, who told me that he was autistic and needed to be tested for fragile X syndrome, which causes mental retardation. We were devastated at this news. We could not control our tears as we prayed to God to have mercy on our son. My husband and I cried together many times during those five weeks before we got the results from the doctor's test. Dr. Devi reassured us that it was his allergies contributing to his behavior. She was kind, confident, and understanding of our pain. She treated me for my emotions; I was an emotional wreck during that time.

When Dr. Devi began eliminating Dominic's food allergy one by one (first one was protein, then milk and calcium, then vitamin C, B complex, sugar, etc.), we began seeing some results. When she treated him for sugar his crying decreased and his head banging ceased. It took two times for him to pass the sugar allergy. He began speaking a few words that made sense to us. He began gesturing for the things he wanted. We continued the treatments and after passing minerals (8th treatment) he began to speak more.

At this time his doctor (specialist) did most of his tests once again. This time we received God's Grace and were told that Dominic's genetic test came back normal. He then started special education classes to help with his speech and fine motor skills. It was then I knew that Dr. Devi's treatments would help bring our son back to us. I was amazed at the progress Dominic had made in such a short time in her office. Now, he is just a happy healthy little boy!

Our older son also has a learning disability and is currently being treated. He also suffered from asthma and sinusitis from childhood. After five basic NAET treatments, Dr. Devi treated him for grasses, pollens, dust, animal epithelium and dander. He can now play in the grass, and cuddle a cat without an asthma attack. He is also showing progress in his learning.

We are very thankful to our friend who shared Dr. Devi's book with me. Otherwise I would have had no way of finding out about this unique treatment. We thank Dr. Devi for her kindness to our family during this time. Thanks to her treatments, our son now lives in "our world." Seeing Dominic's changes, a few other parents have started NAET treatments on their children, and they are also very happy with the results. So many of our children are suffering, I just pray that other doctors who are specializing in treating autistic children, other schools for special education, and parents who have autistic children or who have learning disabilities will find Dr. Devi. I hope they will be encouraged to try the NAET treatments that changed our lives.

Thank you Dr. Devi.

Debbie Lopez, Registered Nurse
Fullerton, CA

(We have come a long way since Debbie Lopez wrote the above for the first edition of this book. Dominic is a straight "A" student, finishing 10th grade now).

NAET Autism Rating Scale

If your child exhibits more than ten of the symptoms from the following list, if you rate them above (2) on each one of them, you should consult a medical specialist to evaluate your child's condition. If any abnormalities are detected, appropriate measures should be taken right away to monitor and treat the condition. The prognosis is better if the treatment is started as soon as the autism is identified. Early detection of autism can give your child the best chance to recover completely.

Interpretation of the NAET Autism Rating Scale

Zero = No allergy related autism

Symptoms 1 to 3 = Mildly allergic

Symptoms 4 to 6 = Moderately Allergic

Symptoms 7 to 10 = Severely Allergic

NAET Autism Rating Scale

Abnormal appetite..............	(0) (1) (2) (3) (4) (5) (6) (7) (8) (9) (10)
Abnormalities in speech.......	(0) (1) (2) (3) (4) (5) (6) (7) (8) (9) (10)
Accident prone.....................	(0) (1) (2) (3) (4) (5) (6) (7) (8) (9) (10)
Aggressive.............................	(0) (1) (2) (3) (4) (5) (6) (7) (8) (9) (10)
Always climbing on objects...	(0) (1) (2) (3) (4) (5) (6) (7) (8) (9) (10)
Appears deaf and/or dumb....	(0) (1) (2) (3) (4) (5) (6) (7) (8) (9) (10)
Biting nails...........................	(0) (1) (2) (3) (4) (5) (6) (7) (8) (9) (10)
Biting own body parts...........	(0) (1) (2) (3) (4) (5) (6) (7) (8) (9) (10)
Bladder problems..................	(0) (1) (2) (3) (4) (5) (6) (7) (8) (9) (10)
Cannot be pacified................	(0) (1) (2) (3) (4) (5) (6) (7) (8) (9) (10)
Cannot determine right from wrong........................	(0) (1) (2) (3) (4) (5) (6) (7) (8) (9) (10)
Cannot tie shoes....................	(0) (1) (2) (3) (4) (5) (6) (7) (8) (9) (10)
Clumsiness............................	(0) (1) (2) (3) (4) (5) (6) (7) (8) (9) (10)
Compulsive touching.............	(0) (1) (2) (3) (4) (5) (6) (7) (8) (9) (10)
Constant motion....................	(0) (1) (2) (3) (4) (5) (6) (7) (8) (9) (10)
Destructive............................	(0) (1) (2) (3) (4) (5) (6) (7) (8) (9) (10)
Dizziness...............................	(0) (1) (2) (3) (4) (5) (6) (7) (8) (9) (10)
Does not ask for help when needed......................	(0) (1) (2) (3) (4) (5) (6) (7) (8) (9) (10)
Eating dirt.............................	(0) (1) (2) (3) (4) (5) (6) (7) (8) (9) (10)
Enuresis (bed wetting)...........	(0) (1) (2) (3) (4) (5) (6) (7) (8) (9) (10)
Erratic disruptive behavior.....	(0) (1) (2) (3) (4) (5) (6) (7) (8) (9) (10)
Excessive drooling.................	(0) (1) (2) (3) (4) (5) (6) (7) (8) (9) (10)
Excessive flatulence...............	(0) (1) (2) (3) (4) (5) (6) (7) (8) (9) (10)
Excessive salivation..............	(0) (1) (2) (3) (4) (5) (6) (7) (8) (9) (10)
Excessive sweating	(0) (1) (2) (3) (4) (5) (6) (7) (8) (9) (10)
Facial changes.......................	(0) (1) (2) (3) (4) (5) (6) (7) (8) (9) (10)
Fat craving.............................	(0) (1) (2) (3) (4) (5) (6) (7) (8) (9) (10)
Fatigued, weak, weary, listless.........................	(0) (1) (2) (3) (4) (5) (6) (7) (8) (9) (10)
Following routines to precise detail...................	(0) (1) (2) (3) (4) (5) (6) (7) (8) (9) (10)

Frequent and repetitive
activity....................................(0) (1) (2) (3) (4) (5) (6) (7) (8) (9) (10)
Frequent burping......................(0) (1) (2) (3) (4) (5) (6) (7) (8) (9) (10)
Frequent flu and colds............. (0) (1) (2) (3) (4) (5) (6) (7) (8) (9) (10)
Greater than normal crying
as an infant.......................... (0) (1) (2) (3) (4) (5) (6) (7) (8) (9) (10)
Growing pains..........................(0) (1) (2) (3) (4) (5) (6) (7) (8) (9) (10)
Hair pulling.............................. (0) (1) (2) (3) (4) (5) (6) (7) (8) (9) (10)
Hand flapping...........................(0) (1) (2) (3) (4) (5) (6) (7) (8) (9) (10)
Head banging........................... (0) (1) (2) (3) (4) (5) (6) (7) (8) (9) (10)
High pain threshold..................(0) (1) (2) (3) (4) (5) (6) (7) (8) (9) (10)
Holds on to people
and objects.......................... (0) (1) (2) (3) (4) (5) (6) (7) (8) (9) (10)
Impaired ability to
role-play............................... (0) (1) (2) (3) (4) (5) (6) (7) (8) (9) (10)
Impaired social play................ (0) (1) (2) (3) (4) (5) (6) (7) (8) (9) (10)
Impaired ability to initiate
speech...............................(0) (1) (2) (3) (4) (5) (6) (7) (8) (9) (10)
Impaired peer relationships.
Impulsive...........................(0) (1) (2) (3) (4) (5) (6) (7) (8) (9) (10)
Increased thirst.
Irritable..............................(0) (1) (2) (3) (4) (5) (6) (7) (8) (9) (10)
Lacks concentration............... (0) (1) (2) (3) (4) (5) (6) (7) (8) (9) (10)
Nightmares.............................. (0) (1) (2) (3) (4) (5) (6) (7) (8) (9) (10)
Loud talk................................. (0) (1) (2) (3) (4) (5) (6) (7) (8) (9) (10)
Muscle aches......................... (0) (1) (2) (3) (4) (5) (6) (7) (8) (9) (10)
Nervous................................... (0) (1) (2) (3) (4) (5) (6) (7) (8) (9) (10)
No eye contact while
communicating....................(0) (1) (2) (3) (4) (5) (6) (7) (8) (9) (10)
Nonstop talk.......................... (0) (1) (2) (3) (4) (5) (6) (7) (8) (9) (10)
Normal or high I.Q.
in certain areas...................(0) (1) (2) (3) (4) (5) (6) (7) (8) (9) (10)
.Not aware of other
people's feelings................ (0) (1) (2) (3) (4) (5) (6) (7) (8) (9) (10)
Onset of unusual activity
in infancy or childhood........(0) (1) (2) (3) (4) (5) (6) (7) (8) (9) (10)
Parrot-like talking................... (0) (1) (2) (3) (4) (5) (6) (7) (8) (9) (10)
Picking at skin, hair, nose........ (0) (1) (2) (3) (4) (5) (6) (7) (8) (9) (10)
Pinches or hurts others............(0) (1) (2) (3) (4) (5) (6) (7) (8) (9) (10)

Poor eye-hand coordination..... (0) (1) (2) (3) (4) (5) (6) (7) (8) (9) (10)
Post nasal drip........................ (0) (1) (2) (3) (4) (5) (6) (7) (8) (9) (10)
Preoccupation with
    parts of objects.................. (0) (1) (2) (3) (4) (5) (6) (7) (8) (9) (10)
Preoccupations in
    narrow interests................. (0) (1) (2) (3) (4) (5) (6) (7) (8) (9) (10)
Protruding abdomen.............. (0) (1) (2) (3) (4) (5) (6) (7) (8) (9) (10)
Puffy below the eyes.............. (0) (1) (2) (3) (4) (5) (6) (7) (8) (9) (10)
Red cheeks........................... (0) (1) (2) (3) (4) (5) (6) (7) (8) (9) (10)
Red earlobes......................... (0) (1) (2) (3) (4) (5) (6) (7) (8) (9) (10)
Restless sleep........................ (0) (1) (2) (3) (4) (5) (6) (7) (8) (9) (10)
Restlessness.......................... (0) (1) (2) (3) (4) (5) (6) (7) (8) (9) (10)
Ring around anus.................... (0) (1) (2) (3) (4) (5) (6) (7) (8) (9) (10)
Rocking................................ (0) (1) (2) (3) (4) (5) (6) (7) (8) (9) (10)
Salt craving........................... (0) (1) (2) (3) (4) (5) (6) (7) (8) (9) (10)
Screaming inconsolably.......... (0) (1) (2) (3) (4) (5) (6) (7) (8) (9) (10)
Self abusive.......................... (0) (1) (2) (3) (4) (5) (6) (7) (8) (9) (10)
Sensitive to cold or heat......... (0) (1) (2) (3) (4) (5) (6) (7) (8) (9) (10)
Sensitive to odors.................. (0) (1) (2) (3) (4) (5) (6) (7) (8) (9) (10)
Sensitive to sound or light...... (0) (1) (2) (3) (4) (5) (6) (7) (8) (9) (10)
Spinning............................... (0) (1) (2) (3) (4) (5) (6) (7) (8) (9) (10)
Spurns affection and cuddling. (0) (1) (2) (3) (4) (5) (6) (7) (8) (9) (10)
Staring at people without
    acknowledgment................ (0) (1) (2) (3) (4) (5) (6) (7) (8) (9) (10)
Sugar craving......................... (0) (1) (2) (3) (4) (5) (6) (7) (8) (9) (10)
Tantrums............................... (0) (1) (2) (3) (4) (5) (6) (7) (8) (9) (10)
Totally nonverbal.................... (0) (1) (2) (3) (4) (5) (6) (7) (8) (9) (10)
Twisting................................ (0) (1) (2) (3) (4) (5) (6) (7) (8) (9) (10)
Uncontrollable
    body movements................ (0) (1) (2) (3) (4) (5) (6) (7) (8) (9) (10)

AUTISM: CHARACTERISTICS AND EFFECTS

WHAT IS AUTISM?

Autism was defined more thoroughly in the introduction of this book, however for a short review: Autism is a syndrome of early childhood; autism is a nutritional deficiency disorder causing biological, neurological and developmental problems in children. The nutritional deficiency is not caused by failing to take enough nutrients by mouth but by poor digestion, absorption, assimilation and utilization of essential nutrients due to allergies. Autistic children are not digesting whatever they consume and their bodies do not receive essential nutrients from food or supplements they take.

The nutritional deficiency will begin to affect the child by the age of three. Usually that is the time most children with regular well-baby checkup visits and appropriate medical care are diagnosed as autistic. Even though the problems resulted from nutritional deficiencies, the developmental problem causes the child to see, feel, smell and hear differently from other people. It is characterized by abnormal social relationships, language disorders with impaired understanding, pronominal reversal (saying you for I or me for you, etc.), rituals such as wiping the face repeatedly, rubbing the nose, pulling hair, chewing long hair constantly, etc., compulsive phenomena and uneven intellectual development, with mental retardation in most cases, if the right treatment is not provided in a timely manner.

The essential nutrients like vitamins, minerals, proteins, starches and fats play a big role in the growth and development stage. If these nutrients are not received in adequate amounts during the growth and development years (first five years of life), the growth and development of various parts of the body and brain are retarded resulting in various abnormalities as we see the symptoms in an autistic child. It prevents individuals from properly understanding what they see and hear. Individuals with autism have extreme difficulty in learning language and social skills and in relating to people. It affects the way the brain uses information because various parts of the brain has not developed properly due to lack of essential factors for the development of the particular tissue. So any of the following factors can affect the brain and cause imbalance in the motor and sensory function as well as other functions: accumulation of certain chemicals in the brain, nuclear radiation, toxins from bacterial and viral infections, toxic exposure from heavy metal, mercury, and silicone; chemically introduced toxins as in vaccination, immunization, etc., genetic factors, food and environmental allergies, also sudden emotional shocks such as witnessing frightful events in childhood, or physical problems affecting those parts of the brain that process language and information. If only one part of the brain is affected from the above listed toxins, then the child will show weakness if the imbalance is in the related tissue or its target organ only. But if more parts or tissues are affected, the child will project all symptoms related to all affected tissues. An autistic child feels isolated from his/her surroundings because he cannot listen to people, he cannot hear any sounds around him, he cannot see properly, he cannot talk, or answer questions because he is not hearing; thus he feels alone in the world isolated from the rest of the people and activities. So he/she finds a way to entertain himself/herself by running in circles, spinning, talking to self and entertaining himself and we call that trait as "Autistic Aloneness". Autism is treatable—early diagnosis and intervention is vital for a good prognosis or outcome.

It is best to consider it as a disability, on a scale from mild to severe. The extreme form of the syndrome may include self-injurious, repetitive, highly unusual and aggressive behavior. Individuals with autism show uneven skill development, with deficits in certain areas, usually in the ability to communicate and relate to others, and distinct skills in other areas. It is important to distinguish autism from mental retardation in which relatively even-skill development is shown. People with autism are not physically disabled and "look" just like anybody without a disability. Because of the invisible nature of autism, it can be much harder to create awareness and understanding of the condition.

In summary, the characteristics of autism vary with each individual and may include the following:

♦ **Delays in Language Development** - Language is slow to develop or it may not develop at all. Individuals who do use language usually have peculiar speech patterns or use words without attaching the normal meaning to them. A monotonal voice is often noted when speech is involved.

♦ **Delays in Social Interactions** - Autistic individuals often avoid eye contact and appear to "tune out the world." There is an impaired ability to develop friendships, understand someone else's feelings or interact and play with peers.

♦ **Variations of Intellectual Functioning** - People with autism may have certain skills that they can excel in, such as music, art, math computation (The Dustin Hoffman character in the movie "Rain Man" is an example), and memorization of facts. Other autistic people may have varying degrees of mental retardation. This combination of intellectual variation makes autism very perplexing to diagnose and treat.

♦ **Compulsive Behavior** - Repetitive body movements, such as twisting, spinning, rocking are common in people with autism. Individuals may repeatedly follow the same route, the same order of dressing, or the same schedule every day. It becomes extremely stressful for autistic individuals if there are changes in their routine.

♦ **Inconsistent Sensory Responses** - Sometimes people identified as autistic may appear deaf and fail to respond to words or other sounds. At other times they may be distressed by an everyday noise, like a dog barking. There also may be a tendency to be insensitive to pain, unresponsive to heat or cold or they may overreact to any of these.

The above described characteristics have been observed and documented by the pioneers who specialized in diagnosing autism. Unfortunately, no one seemed to explore the underlying causes. I have treated many autistic children in my allergy practice and have received phenomenal results by simply eliminating their allergies to the foods, fabrics, chemicals, and environmental toxins they come in contact with in their daily lives. I have found specific allergic patterns and reactions behind autistic behaviors.

HISTORY OF AUTISM

Leo Kanner and Hans Asperger were the first to publish accounts of childhood autism. Working independently, Kanner in Baltimore (1943), and Asperger in Vienna (1944), detailed case studies and attempted to describe the disorder. Before Leo Kanner wrote his paper identifying autistic children, these children were classified as emotionally disturbed or mentally retarded. Kanner observed that the children were not merely slow learners, they didn't fall in the category of emotionally disturbed. He presented 11 children in his study whose behaviors were so different from anything he had noticed previously that he felt they needed a new category, which he called *Early Infantile Autism*. He noted certain features which are discernible in all true cases of autism: *autistic aloneness* which refers to the child disregarding or ignoring anything from the outside environment, *desire for sameness* such as repetitive motions and noises, and *islets of ability* such as the ability to recollect poems, complex patterns, and sequences which represent good intelligence.

Asperger gave detailed descriptions of autistic children. He found that they all had common fundamental disturbances in their social integration. However, he also felt that they had an originality of thought and experience, which might lead them to exceptional achievement as they grow older. He also noted that autistic children's language was unnatural; they followed their own impulses and had many stereotypical movements along with a narrow area of intellectual ability. The patients Asperger identified all had speech, so the term Asperger's Syndrome is used to label autistic people with speech, at the higher functioning end of the autism spectrum, while Kanner's Syndrome is used for the classical, limited speech and low functioning, form of autism.

Before Leo Kanner and Hans Asperger described autism to the world through their published works, a Swiss psychiatrist, Eugenc Bleuler had already introduced the word autism in a 1912 edition of *The American Journal of Insanity.* Bleuler is particularly notable for naming schizophrenia, a disorder which was previously known as *dementia praecox.* Bleuler realised the condition was neither a dementia, nor did it always occur in young people (praecox meaning early) and so gave the condition the name from the Greek for split (schizo) and mind (phrene). He originally used the word autism to refer to a basic disturbance in schizophrenia, the narrowing of relationships to people and the outside world. The narrowing became so extreme in autism, it excluded everything except the person's own self. This word also comes from the Greek word *autos* meaning self.

THE IMMUNE SYSTEM, ALLERGY, AND AUTISM

CHARACTERISTICS OF AUTISM

Even though the immune system is only a part of a larger hormonal and neurochemical control system, it plays a huge role in supervising and maintaining the body and its various body functions in appropriate manner. It demands proper fuel for its function from daily intake of nutrients. If the body (along with the immune system) is heavily engaged in combating invaders, and if the function of acceptance and assimilation of nutrients are ignored, the immune system will be left without the fuel for further function. This weakens the immune system further, leaving the person fatigued. In this weakened state, we are also more vulnerable to bacterial or viral infections because our finite immune defenses are preoccupied with combating or neutralizing the foreign substances; they are too tired to carry out the protective function.

COMBINING PAST AND PRESENT MEDICAL PRACTICES

Allergic manifestations can be seen as the following in sensitive people: itching, rashes, hives, ear infections, edema, asthma, joint pains, muscle aches, headaches, restlessness, insomnia, addictions, craving, indigestion, vomiting, anger, depression, disturbed vision, incontinence, repeated infections, panic attacks, brain fatigue, learning disability, dyslexia, and brain fog. Most children seem to have inherited allergic tendencies from their ancestors. They may have allergic reactions to foods, chemicals, environmental factors, even the people they come in contact with in everyday life. In an autistic person, the allergies affect the different parts of the brain and cause delayed language development, delay in social interactions, variations in intellectual ability, compulsive behaviors, and inconsistent sensory responses.

Presently we have limited understanding of the human brain and its functions when evaluated through Western perspectives. Medical science is looking for ways to understand the functions of the brain and prove theories through scientific means. We might wait a long time to find all the answers to our questions, since we only have knowledge of about 10 percent of human brain function. Until the other 90 percent is explored, we may not have the answers we are looking for. While waiting for solid answers, many of us may miss the boat.

On the other hand, 5,000 years ago, Oriental medicine explored the functions of the human body and brain and understood them enough to solve many health disorders in order to help make living easier. Oriental medical pioneers did this without cutting cadavers, but by studying living persons. It may not sound totally scientific, but for centuries Oriental medicine has helped millions upon millions of people understand their problems in order to assist them to live better lives. If we take Oriental medical principles into consideration, which deal with cause and solution, we could live our lives more normally. If we find the cause, elimination can be relatively easy with the help of NAET.

POSSIBLE CAUSES OF AUTISM

When I evaluated autistic children (and adults) through Oriental medical principles, I saw certain typical patterns of energy disturbances in certain energy meridians or pathways. Most of the autistic children I have seen suffered from energy disturbances in the Kidney, Liver, Spleen, Stomach, Heart, and Small Intestine meridians.

♦ Kidney meridian disturbance can produce inherited allergic tendencies.

♦ Liver meridian disturbance can produce allergy to chemicals and the environment. This also produces anger, temper tantrums, irritability, stereotypical behaviors like hand flapping, hair pulling and other repeated body movements, auto-stimulation, etc.

♦ Spleen meridian disturbance can cause speech disorders like a delay in speech, abnormal speech, abnormal or poor social interaction, delay in language development, variation of intellectual abilities, and craving sweets. The disturbance in this meridian also causes autistic loneliness.

♦ Disturbance in the small intestine, liver and kidney meridians can cause inconsistent sensory responses.

♦ Disturbance in the stomach meridian can cause aggressive behaviors, voracious appetite or poor appetite. (Please read Chapter Seven on acupuncture meridians for more information on symptoms and the meridian connection.)

An allergic predisposition or tendency is inherited, but the allergy itself may not manifest until some later date. Researchers have found that when both parents were or are allergy-sensitive, 75 to 100 percent of their offspring react to those same allergens. When neither of the parents is (was) sensitive to allergens, the probability of producing allergic offspring drops dramatically to less than 10 percent. Most of us suffer from allergic manifestations in varying degrees, because of the different levels of our parental inheritance.

Studies have shown that, in some cases, even when parents had no allergies, their offspring still suffered from many allergies since birth. In these cases, various possibilities exist:

♦ The parents may have suffered from a serious disease or condition. For example, the parents had rheumatic fever before the child was born, which caused an alteration in the genetic codes.

♦ The pregnant mother may have been exposed to harmful substances such as:

radiation - X-rays,

chemicals - such as an expectant mother taking too much caffeine, alcohol, and exposure to chemicals such as carbon monoxide poisoning,

circulating internal toxins - as the result of a disease, for instance streptococcal infection as in strep-throat, measles, chicken pox, candidiasis, parasitic infestation and diabetes.

drug-induced toxins which may be the result of allergic reactions.

allergic reactions to vaccinations, immunizations, antibiotics, other drugs,

emotional trauma such as the sudden loss of loved ones, various kinds of abuses like mental torture, rape, fearful events like a major fire in the living quarters, falls, etc.

The parents may have suffered severe malnutrition, by not getting enough food or not assimilating food due to poor absorption caused by allergies. Thus possibly causing the growing embryo to undergo cell mutation during its development in the womb. The altered cells do not carry over the original genetic codes or do not go through normal development. The organs and tissues that are supposed to develop from the affected cells have impaired function.

In our modern life, many parents leave their infants in front of a color television permitting the infant to bathe in a continuous flow of radiation for hours. Excess assimilation of television radiation can cause energy blockages and cell mutation in the growing infant.

A study published in 2003 that followed about 2,600 children from birth to age seven found that serious attention problems can result from children watching TV. In addition, the study found that brain abnormalities can result, the younger the child, the more serious the problems. The American Academy of Pediatrics recommends no TV, no videos, no computer games before age two.

Our ancestors were not exposed to these new technologies, chemicals and pollutants because this explosion happened unexpectedly with the scientific advancement at the dawn of the 21st Century.

Our genes were thrown rather suddenly into the midst of the newly created chemicals and environmental pollutants. They did not have enough time to prepare themselves to evolve gradually and to add the new information into their memory banks, in order to live appropriately in our present environment. We call ourselves healthy when our genes are able to recognize the things around us and respond appropriately, without causing any dysfunction in the body. In a healthy state, we are able to tolerate the substances we eat or the environment and chemicals we are exposed to. But, when we inherit genes that are not prepared appropriately to face the present world, they do not recognize the new changes around us. Due to the sudden transition, some of these genes remain hypoactive (dormant) towards the surroundings and others become hyperactive not knowing the right thing to do. In either case, both do not function normally.

When genes do not recognize certain substances in their environment appropriately, they panic and begin generating adverse reactions in the body of the bearer, which we call "allergies." For our purpose, an allergy is defined as an adverse reaction of one individual to a substance from his/her environment that may be harmless or beneficial to another individual. From this definition of allergy came the familiar phrase, "one man's meat is another man's poison." An allergic reaction may be manifested in varying degrees as mild to severe. Irritability (hypo or hyper reaction) of the brain and nervous system leads to inappropriate functioning of the body, mind and spirit. When the reactions are hypo, the interaction between the person and the substance from the environment produces little to no response at all. When the person produces a hyper reaction towards certain things, the body perceives these foreign substances as a threat to its safety and survival, the immune system is activated and the defenses against the invaders are brought in. When the body engages in the battle against foreign invaders, the body becomes very sensitive, the immune system, defense center, repair center, and maintenance systems divert themselves to combating the invaders. This means that they defer repair until the immediate perceived assault of foreign exposure is over.

NAET is a non-invasive method that can identify, treat and eliminate the adverse reactions of the genes to any allergens, including the new, unfamiliar substances. This treatment will gently introduce the new substances from one's surroundings to the misinformed genes. When the genes get formally introduced through NAET treatments to all substances from one's surroundings, genes do not get confused with future contacts with the formally intoduced substances, thus preventing the body from having allergies and allergy-related disorders, including allergy-related autism.

NAET: COMBINING THE BEST OF EAST AND WEST

WHAT IS NAET?

Nambudripad's Allergy Elimination Techniques, or NAET, is an integrative medical approach. NAET was developed from Oriental medicine, chiropractic techniques and nutritional discipline. Nambudripad's Testing Procedure (NTP) uses Oriental medical principles to evaluate a patient's health condition. Standard medical diagnostic procedures are used to support Oriental medical diagnostic findings. In 1983, I originated NAET to eliminate food and environmental allergic reactions, to balance the unbalanced energies, to remove the adverse reaction of foreign energies and make them compatible with the body, successfully restoring normal body functions, applying simple chiropractic and acupuncture principles, manipulating the 31 pairs of spinal nerve roots and associated sympathetic and parasympathetic nerve fibers.

Through many years of research, and after many trials and errors, NAET is developed to permanently eliminate energy disturbances in the energy pathways caused from allergies. These energy disturbance elimination techniques together are called Nambudripad's Allergy Elimination Techniques or NAET for short.

NAET uses Chiropractic principles to administer the treatments. Post treatment health is maintained using nutritional principles. With the help of NTP, the patient's immune system status, the intensity of the condition, the associated meridians and the related nerve root(s) are determined. Then the causative agent is determined from the list of "major categories of causative factors of disease" given in chapter two. A substance(s) or a factor(s) from these groups may cause an energy imbalance in the respective energy meridian(s) causing autistic behaviors. That particular substance – an allergen – is determined as the cause.

The symptoms, diagnosis and treatment of sensitivities, hypersensitivities and intolerances, and allergies often overlap. Both intolerances and allergies, in varying degrees, can be tested by Neuromuscular Sensitivity Testing (NST) by producing a weak NST, weakness of the indicator muscle in the case of an allergy, or a strong NST, strong resistance by the indicator muscle, in the case of no allergy. All of these allergic reactions are capable of producing autism, and can successfully be treated by NAET.

ALLOPATHY AND WESTERN SCIENCE

Knowledge of the brain, cranial nerves, spinal nerves, and autonomic nervous system from Western medicine enlightens us about the body's efficient multilevel communication network. Through this network of nerves, vital energy circulates in the body carrying negative and positive messages from each and every cell to the brain and then back to the cells. A cell or tissue sends one message to the brain. The brain sends out the reply in a matter of nanoseconds to the rest of the body. Knowledge about the nervous system, its origin, travel route, and the organs and tissues that benefit from its nerve energy supply (target organs and tissues), helps us to understand the energy distribution of the spinal nerves emerging from the 31 pairs of spinal nerve roots. [6]

KINESIOLOGY

Kinesiology is the art and science of movement of the human body. Kinesiology is used in NAET to compare the strength and weakness of any muscle of the body in the presence or absence of any substance. This is called Neuromuscular Sensitivity Testing (NST). NST is slightly different from MRT. In NST, balancing the energy meridians is involved to achieve accurate result in detecting allergies. It may not be necessary in simple Muscle Response Testing (MRT). It is hypothesized that this measurable weakness of a particular muscle is produced by the generation of an energy obstruction in the particular spinal nerve route that corresponds to the weakened muscle when the specific item is in its energy field. Any item that is capable of producing energy obstruction in any spinal nerve route is called an *allergen*. Through this simple kinesiological testing method, allergens can be detected, obstructed spinal nerves and their routes, and the affected organs, tissues, and other body parts can be identified.

CHIROPRACTIC

Chiropractic technique helps us to detect the nerve energy blockage in a specific nerve energy pathway by detecting and isolating the exact nerve root that is being pinched. The exact vertebral level in relation to the pinched spinal nerve root helps us to trace the travel route, the destination, and the target organs of that particular energy pathway. Chiropractic medicine postulates that a pinched nerve or any such disturbance in the energy flow can cause disease in the target organ, stressing the importance of maintaining an uninterrupted flow of nerve energy. A pinched nerve, or an obstruction in the energy flow, can result from an allergy. Spinal manipulation at the specific vertebral level of the pinched nerve can relieve the obstruction of the energy flow and help the body come to a state of homeostasis (i.e. a state of perfect balance between the body and all surrounding energies and their functions).

ACUPUNCTURE/ORIENTAL MEDICINE

Yin-Yang theory from Oriental medical principles also teaches the importance of maintaining homeostasis or balance in the body. According to Oriental medical principles, "when the Yin and Yang are balanced in the body (a state of perfect balance between all energies and functions), no disease is possible." Any disturbance in the homeostasis can cause disease. Any allergen that is capable of producing a weakening effect of the muscles in the body can cause disturbance in the homeostasis. By isolating and eliminating the cause of the disturbance, in this case an allergen, and by maintaining an absolute homeostasis, diseases can be prevented and cured. According to acupuncture theory, acupuncture and/or acupressure at certain acupuncture points is capable of bringing the body into a state of homeostasis, by removing the energy disturbances from the twelve (meridian) energy pathways. When the energy disturbances are removed, energy can flow freely through the energy meridians bringing the body into a perfect balance.

NUTRITION

You are what you eat! The secret to good health is achieved through correct nutrition. What is correct nutrition? How do you get it? When you can eat nutritious foods without discomfort and assimilate the nutrients from the food, that food is the right food for you. When you get indigestion, bloating, other digestive troubles, constipation, diarrhea, depression, hyperactivity, mood swings, anger, insomnia, sleepiness, fatigue, poor concentration, diminished clarity of thinking, brain fog, pain in the joints and muscles, nervousness, heart palpitation, itching anywhere in the body upon or after eating a particular food, that food is not helping you to function normally. Regardless of how natural, expensive, or packed with high quality nutrition, if a food item causes one or more of these symptoms upon ingestion, it is not the right nutrition for you. This is due to an allergy to that food. Different people react differently to the same food. So, it is very important to clear the allergy to the nutrients in the food. For this reason, allergic people can tolerate food that is low in nutrition better than nutritious food. After clearing the allergy, you should try to eat more wholesome, nutritious foods. Above all, you should avoid refined, bleached foods devoid of nutrients.

Many people who feel poorly due to undiagnosed food allergies may take vitamins or other supplements to increase their vitality. This can actually make them feel worse if they happen to be allergic to these nutrients as well. Only after clearing those allergies can their bodies assimilate them properly.

NAET involves the whole brain and its network of nerves as it reprograms the brain by erasing a previous harmful memory regarding an allergen, and imprinting a new useful memory in its place. To comprehend NAET, some understanding of the brain and its functions is necessary. Many books on the subject of the brain are available in bookstores and libraries. For more information, please consult the references in the bibliography.

INCOMPATIBILITIES / IMBALANCES

The energy blockages in the human body are caused by incompatible electromagnetic charges around the body. When there is an incompatible charge around the body, there is an altered reaction in the body. Energy incompatibilities that are capable of producing various ailments are used synonymously with *allergy* in this book.

When we talk about health conditions, there is hardly a human disease or condition that may not involve an allergic factor; autism spectrum disorders are not any different. Any portion of the body, organ, or group of organs may be involved, though the allergic responses may vary greatly from one item to another and from one person to another.

Major illnesses, severe reactions to foods, drinks, drugs, bacterial toxins, chemicals, radiation, emotional stresses, etc., are capable of causing damage to the central and autonomic nerve fibers thus inhibiting their conductivity. This poor conductivity causes allergy and allergy-related illnesses.

The brain, through 31 pairs of spinal nerves, operates the best network of communication ever known. Energy blockages take place in a person's body due to contact with adverse energy of other substances. When two adverse energies come close, repulsion takes place. When two compatible energies come together, attraction takes place.

This enhances the supply of adequate nutrients to the brain. When the brain receives sufficient nutrients it can function normally and coordinate the rest of the body to carry out the body functions appropriately. When the brain is not coordinating with the vital organs, physiological functions are impaired. When the circulation of the energy is restored in the energy pathways, the vital organs resume their routine work and function properly. The brain and body together, will remove any toxic buildup through the body's natural excretory mechanisms.

Certain parts of the body get diminished energy and nutrient supply, when the central, sympathetic, and parasympathetic nerves are not coordinating well, thus causing improper energy circulation. When this happens, the weakest part of the body fails first. If the weakest part of the body happens to be the brain, or any part of the brain, and if the energy supply to the brain is reduced or stopped, abnormalities or poor functions of the brain are seen. Then a person may demonstrate autistic disorders, manic depressive disorders, schizophrenic, and other neurological disorders, all due to lack of energy and nutrient supply to the brain. This can be tested and demonstrated by various equipment and devices such as: E.E.G (electroencephalogram), EDS (electrodermal screening), and HRV (reading of autonomic system balance).

NAET can remove the energy interferences in the energy pathways and restart normal energy circulation through the brain and nervous system.

Over eight thousand medical professionals world-wide have been trained to treat their patients with NAET. Regular training sessions are being conducted several times a year to prepare many more licensed medical professionals to meet the challenge. This book will educate individuals concerning the treatment, and in some cases, to test themselves or their children to locate the cause of their problems.

The information about the NAET training available for licensed medical practitioners can be obtained from our website **www.naet.com**   or by contacting us:

NAET Central Office
6714 Beach Blvd.
Buena Park, CA 90621
Tel: 1-714-523- 8900
Fax: 1-714-523-3068
E-mail: naet@earthlink.net

Say Good-bye to Allergy-related Autism

2

ALLERGY RELATED AUTISM

We are discussing allergy-related autism in this book. There are hardly any human diseases or conditions in which allergic factors are not involved directly or indirectly. Autism is not any different. Any substance under the sun, including sunlight itself, can cause an allergic reaction in susceptible individuals. In other words, you can potentially be allergic to anything you come in contact with. If you begin to check children around you—not only children with autism, even so called healthy children—you will find them reacting to many things around them.

But every one reacts differently to allergens. There is no single type of reaction that can be recognized in every allergic person to a particular allergen. You can be allergic to: foods, drinks, drugs, childhood immunizations, herbs, vitamins, water, clothing, jewelry, cold, heat, wind, food colors, additives, preservatives, chemicals, formaldehyde etc. Undiagnosed allergies can produce symptoms of various health disorders including autism.

When the patient's diagnosis is correct, results are less frightening than if undetected. By learning the simple Nambudripad's Testing Procedures (NTP), anyone, professional or layman, can easily learn to recognize various allergens and the symptoms they cause. This will help you begin to seek the appropriate diagnostic studies and pursue proper health care as needed.

Science and technology have altered the life-style of humankind enormously. The reactions and diseases arising from responses to these technological changes are very different. Our quality of life has improved with these scientific achievements. Yet, these same scientific accomplishments have become everlasting nightmares for people suffering from autism.

Over time, technology is becoming more pervasive in every aspect of life. Let's face it; technology will always be with us. However, people with autism and other related neurological disorders, must find ways to overcome adverse reactions to the new chemicals and other allergens they are exposed to, created by new technology. NAET fits right in with the 21st century life-style. Nambudripad's Allergy Elimination Treatments (NAET) which requires a series of detailed treatments, and NTP offer the prospect of relief to people who suffer from allergies, whether caused by technological advances or other factors.

Behavioral and Physical Characteristics of Autism

•   Communication difficulties: nonverbal, repeats what is said, no response to "stop" command, runs or moves away, covers ears, and looks away constantly.

•   May appear argumentative, stubborn, belligerent, may incessantly ask "Why?" or answers "No" to all questions.

•   Will have difficulty interpreting body language, and facial expressions, jokes, and teasing.

•   May be poor listeners, may not seem to care what others have to say, may lack eye contact.

•   May have passive monotonal voices with incorrect and/or unusual pronunciations, often sounds like a computer generated robot.

•   Difficulty in judging personal space: may stand too close or too far away, may stare at people, sometimes coming too close to the face.

•   May persevere on topics that interest them, may repeatedly ask the same questions about their area of interest. They may not see another person's point of view

•   They are very honest, perhaps too honest, and not tactful.

•   They may not: recognize danger, differentiate between minor or major problems, know how and where to get help, be able to give answers to questions.

•   May have candida, yeast problems, parasite infestation, chronic fatigue, immune disorders, hormonal imbalances, ear infections, and pediatric problems.

•   May have digestive disorders, anxiety disorders, various other mental disorders, depression, and various emotional imbalances, etc.

•   Other symptoms include circulatory disorders, sleep irregularity, chemical sensitivity, nutritional disorders, restless leg syndrome, skin ailments, and genitourinary disorders.

All of the above symptoms may be due to allergy. When these affect certain parts of the brain in allergic children, they exhibit autistic symptoms. Each child should be evaluated separately for the allergies, reactions, and areas that are affected by a particular allergen. Autistic children react to allergens differently than most people, and exhibit different symptoms. There are no typical responses to allergens in the real world. If medical practitioners are depending on allergies to produce a uniform set of responses for all people, they may misdiagnose and thereby provide the wrong treatment.

CATEGORIES OF ALLERGENS

Common allergens are generally classified into nine basic categories; based primarily on the method of exposure, rather than the symptoms they produce. In a child with autism the first organ in the body that is affected is the brain and the typical symptoms of brain allergy are exhibited. The nine categories of allergens are:

1. Inhalants are those allergens that are contacted through the nose, throat and bronchial tubes. Examples of inhalants are microscopic spores, of certain grasses, flowers, pollens, powders, smoke, cosmetics, perfumes, different aromas including food-cooking odors, chemical fumes such as paint, varnish, pesticides, insecticides, fertilizers, flour from grains, etc.

2. Ingestants are allergens which are contacted through the mouth and find their way into the gastrointestinal tract. These include foods, condiments, drugs, beverages, chewing gum, vitamin supplements, food colorings, food additives, etc. We must not ignore the potential reactions to things that are touched, and then inadvertently transmitted into the mouth through our hands.

The area of ingested allergens is one of the most difficult to diagnose because the allergic responses are often delayed from several minutes to several days

3. Contactants produce their effect by direct contact with the skin; they include: environmental allergens, fabrics, bed linen, night-wares, pillow, stuffed toys, toys, furniture, books, coloring books, coloring materials, arts and craft items, school bag, cats, dogs, rabbits, cosmetics, soaps, skin creams, detergents, rubbing alcohol, latex gloves, hair dyes, various types of plant oils, and chemicals such as gasoline, dyes, acrylic nails, nail polish, fabrics, formaldehyde, etc.

4. Injectants are allergens injected into the skin, muscles, joints and blood vessels in the form of various serums, antitoxins, vaccines, childhood immunizations, and drugs. Injectants also include substances entering the body through insect bites.

5. Infectants are allergens that produce their effect by causing sensitivity to an infectious agent, such as a virus or bacteria. For example, an allergic reaction may result when tuberculin bacterium is introduced as part of a diagnostic test to determine a patient's sensitivity or reaction to it.

6. Physical Agents include: heat, humid air, cold, cold mist, sun radiation, dampness, drafts, changes in barometric pressure, high altitude, carbon dioxide, carbon monoxide, air conditioning; other types of radiation like computer, microwave, X-ray, geopathic radiation, electrical and electromagnetic radiation, fluorescent lights, radiation from cellular and cordless telephones, and radiation from power lines are irritants. Mechanical irritants include: vibrations from a washer and dryer, hair dryer, electric shaver, massager, motion vibrations from a moving automobile, motion sickness (car sickness, sea sickness), sickness while playing sports, roller coaster rides and/or horseback riding. Sounds causing allergic reactions include: airplanes, traffic noises, loud music and voices in a particular pitch. All of the above are known as physical allergens. Burns may also be included in this category.

7. Genetic Factors are tendencies toward allergies carried over from parents and grandparents. Allergies can also skip generations or manifest differently in parents than in their children.

8. Molds and Fungi are in a category by themselves because of the numerous avenues through which they can come into contact with people in everyday life. They can be ingested, inhaled, touched, or even (as in the case of penicillin) injected. They can also come in the form of airborne spores making up a large part of the dust we breathe and pick up in our vacuum cleaners, in fluids such as our drinking water, and the dark fungal growth, in the corners of damp rooms. They can appear on the body as athlete's foot and in particular fetid vaginal conditions, commonly called "yeast infections." Molds and fungi also grow on trees and in the damp soil, and are sources of: food (truffles and mushrooms), disease (ringworm and the aforementioned yeast infections), and even of medicine (penicillin). Many autistic children suffer from yeast, candida, mold, and fungus overgrowth in the body. Most mothers of autistic children have the history of vaginal yeast infection during pregnancy.

9. Emotional Factors can affect children who become autistic later. Sudden fears, frightening sights, etc. can give sudden shock to the child's brain and later cause autism-like symptoms.

INHALANTS

It is typical for a person with autism to react to most of these environmental allergens. The symptoms of a person with autism arising from the interactions with inhaled allergens varies greatly from a typical response of an environmentally sensitive person. In a child with autism the first organ in the body that is affected is the brain and the typical symptoms of brain allergy are exhibited.

INGESTANTS

Ingestion makes the direct association between cause and effect very difficult. Some people can react violently in seconds after they consume an allergen. In extreme cases, just touching or coming near the allergen is enough to forewarn the central nervous system that it is about to be poisoned, resulting in a premature allergic reaction (an anaphylactic shock). Usually more violent reactions are observed in ingested allergens than in any other forms. The area of ingested allergens is one of the most difficult to diagnose because the allergic responses are often delayed from several minutes to several days. This makes the direct association between cause and effect very difficult.

Such was the case of 4-year-old Austin, who doubled over or rolled over on the ground and cried every time he ate any food. He became very irritable at times. He just rocked back and forth in his chair, or ran in circles nonstop until he got tired. He was becoming antisocial, refusing to meet other children and/or go out and play with them.

He was referred to us by a family friend. Austin was examined using NTP. He was found to be allergic to all the 30 groups of foods from the basic NAET list, and many from the environmental groups. His mother had the history of yeast infection off and on throughout her pregnancy. She also had gestational diabetes. These two symptoms we have noted in most mothers of children with autism and ADHD.

Austin's treatments progressed slowly. He was highly allergic to egg white, vitamin C, milk casein, tyramine, lactic acid, wheat, gluten, gliadin, sugar mix, mineral mix, salt mix, food colorings, tomato, pesticides, formaldehyde, and MMR (immunization). He craved salt. He enjoyed eating salt by itself whenever he got some in his hands. His mother kept the salt in the cabinet and kept it under lock all the time. His favorite snack was pretzels with salt crystals on them. Many autistic individuals crave salt. According to Oriental medicine, these individuals have huge kidney meridian imbalances causing poor digestion and assimilation of sodium chloride causing them to crave.

Austin's strange behavior and stomach ache came under control when he passed the treatment for salt, and gliadin, one of the natural substances seen in wheat. We continued to treat him for all known other allergens which tested weak by NST - almost 65 groups. He appeared cheerful, became focused, attentive, and friendly by the time he was ready for school.

We live in a highly technological age. New substances are being introduced into our diets to preserve color, flavor, and to extend the shelf life of our foods. There are some additives used in foods as preservatives that have caused severe health problems. Some artificial sweeteners cause mysterious problems in particular people. They may mimic symptoms of serious disorders (autism, ADHD and other brain disorders, etc.). Clinical depression, antisocial behaviors, itching, hives, confusion, insomnia, and vertigo, can also be reactions from an allergy to food coloring and/or preservatives. The majority of these additives are harmless to most people, but can be disabling and life-threatening to those who react to them.

Great care must be taken to know exactly what is contained in anything a person with allergies puts into his/her mouth. If everyone could become proficient in NST, by using this simple testing before eating foods, most hazardous reactions from food allergies could be prevented. (Read Chapter 6 for more information on NST).

CONTACTANTS

Allergic reactions to contactants can be different in each person, and sensitive children may exhibit symptoms of autism.

Various natural or synthetic fabrics can affect autistic children and adults. Many children react to cotton even though it is a natural fiber. Cotton is used in numerous items. It is not easy to find a fabric that is made from only one type of material anymore. Many products seen in shops are a blend of many things. Cotton fibers are used in carpets, elastics, bed sheet, fleece material, cosmetic applicators, toilet paper, paper towels, etc. Wool may also cause brain imbalances in sensitive persons. Some people, who are sensitive to wool, also react to creams with a lanolin base since lanolin is derived from sheep wool. Some people can be allergic to cotton socks, nylon socks or woolen socks, causing them to have abnormal behaviors. Children can also be allergic to carpets, drapes and ceramic tiles or marbles, and these items can cause adverse reactions in sensitive children.

A lot of children are allergic to crude oils, plant oils and their derivatives, which include plastic and synthetic rubber products as well as latex products. Many children react to their favorite toys or teddy huggers. Can you imagine the difficulty of living in this modern society, and attempting to be completely free from products made of crude oil? A person would literally be immobilized. The phones we use, the milk containers we drink from, the polyester fabrics we wear, most of the face and body creams we use... all are made from a common product – crude oil!

Food items normally classified as ingestants—may also act as contactants on persons who over time handle them constantly. They can cause migraines, headaches, brain irritability, anger, temper tantrums, fatigue, brain fog, confusion, crying spells, mood swings, insomnia, depression, etc.

One can be allergic to cooking smells, smells from cleaning agents, paper products, paper bags, plastic bags, ink, pens, pencils, plants, fertilizers, crayons, etc. One can also be allergic to toilet paper, and currency bills. Care must be taken to isolate the allergen efficiently so that precise treatment can be provided.

INJECTANTS

Allergens are injected into the skin, muscles, joints and blood vessels in the form of various serums, antitoxins, vaccines, childhood immunizations, and drugs. Injectants also include substances entering the body through insect bites. As with any other allergic reaction, the injection of a sensitive drug into the system creates the risk of producing dangerous allergic reactions. To the sensitive person, the drug actively becomes a poison with the same effect as an injection of arsenic. The seemingly harmless substance can become more allergenic for certain people over time, without the person being aware of the potential risk. For example, take the increasing number of incidents of allergies to the drug penicillin. The reactions vary and include: hives, diarrhea, and in more severe cases anaphylactic shock and/or death.

Various vaccinations and immunizations may also produce allergic reactions. I have noted in the history of most autistic children, even though they had lots of minor allergies since birth, they were normal in their growth and development before they reached 18 months or so. Then they began showing different health and behavioral disorders. Some parents could trace their children's behavioral changes beginning from reactions to antibiotics and booster doses of immunizations. While receiving their usual immunizations, many children become extremely ill physically, physiologically, and emotionally. Some children do not exhibit any immediate reactions. If the children were allergic to the injected vaccine, if they did not exhibit any immediate symptoms, they could have a delayed reaction.

How does the delayed reaction take place? It can be explained easily by Oriental medical theory. The child is allergic to the substance, but it is mild and initially causes energy disturbance in one or two meridians only. If the body cannot resolve the energy disturbance in a few hours, because of the Yin-Yang relationships of the meridians, eventually other meridians will get involved. Eventually, the energy disturbance will spread through all 12 meridians and begin to develop reactions in deeper levels. Various neurological disorders, hyperactive disorders, attention deficit disorders, mental retardation, manic disorders, Crohn's disease, chronic irritable bowel syndrome, tumors, and cysts, etc., may develop as a delayed reaction of a childhood immunization.

Before injection, every item can be checked using NST and if found weak, it should not be injected, or at least it should be postponed until it is desensitized with NAET. Great care must be taken before giving immunizations to children. Items should be screened using NST before injecting the child with any immunizations. It is also advisable to inject one drug at a time instead of mixing up three or four vaccines in one session. Some nonallergic children may be able to tolerate the vaccine mix. But children with an allergic history should not receive multiple vaccines in one session.

Why do most children get excess reaction after 18 months? Usually, the primary injection (usually given before 6 months of age) may not cause severe reactions in children. In an allergic person, with the first exposure, the immune system is alerted; with the second or third exposure, the already alerted immune system goes into action giving rise to reactions with different intensities. However, even after the reaction has started, if NAET is administered correctly and immediately, it can stop severe damage to the system, or reverse the reaction and restore the function.

Sometimes a combined reaction produces more damage than a reaction from a single source. When children react to immunizations, many of them get a fever and upper respiratory infections, cough, bronchitis, etc., if they are allergic to vaccinations and/or immunization drugs. These symptoms are usually treated with antibiotics. If the child is also allergic to antibiotics, the child has to fight two allergens independently in addition to fighting the combined reaction. This causes the child to fight three reactions at the same time and the weakest part of the body gives up first. All these toxins can easily cross the blood-brain barrier and affect the brain.

Such was the case of a 5-year-old boy Daniel, who became very sick after a regular MMR booster dose. He had a continuous fever (102 degrees Fahrenheit) that lasted for six weeks. Finally, when the fever came down to a normal level, he became irritable, aggressive, short tempered, and antisocial. He couldn't play with other children without kicking, hitting, biting or spitting on them. He talked constantly and craved sweets all the time. He ran around the house playing hide and seek in the middle of the night instead of sleeping. His worried parents brought him to see me. His problem was traced to the MMR immunization, after testing with NTP. He was treated for all the basics and MMR vaccine with NAET, after which he became well again.

INFECTANTS

A typical reaction to the tuberculin test may be seen as an infectious eruption under the skin. This type of reaction may occur with a skin patch or scratch tests performed in the normal course of allergy testing by the traditional medical approach.

Infectants differ from injectants because of the nature of the allergic substance; that is a substance, which is a known injectant and is limited in the amount administered to the patient. A slight prick of the skin introduces the toxin through the epidermis and a pox, or similar harmless skin lesion will erupt if the patient is allergic to that substance. For most people, the pox soon dries up and forms a scab that eventually heals, without much discomfort. However, in some cases the site of the injectant becomes infected and the usual inflammatory process can be seen (heat, redness, swelling, pain, drainage of pus from the site for many days).

In other words, the introduction of an allergen into a reactive person's system creates the potential risk of causing a severe response regardless of the amount of the toxic substance used.

The brain and parts of the brain can get affected and cause autism, ADHD, etc. Every one of the autistic children I have treated had a history of taking antibiotics for reactions following immunizations. The antibiotics should be screened by NST for any possible allergies alone or in combination, before administering to the child. The prescribing doctor, the administering pharmacist, nurse and the parents should learn

NST to screen antibiotics before administration. **Prevention is always better than a cure.**

It should be noted that bacteria and virus are contacted in numerous ways. Our casual contact with objects and people expose us to dangerous contaminants and possible illnesses daily. When our autoimmune systems are functioning properly, we pass off the illness without notice. It is when our systems are not working at maximum performance levels that we experience infections, fevers, and other discomforts. Children with autism should not be allowed to come in contact with other people who suffer from infections like upper respiratory infections, flu virus, and bacterial infections.

PHYSICAL AGENTS

When the patient suffers from more than one allergy, physical agents can affect the patient greatly. If the child has already eaten an allergic food item, then walks in the cold air, he might develop upper respiratory problems, a sore throat, asthma or joint pains, etc., depending on the organ or meridian affected. Heat, humid air, cold, cold mist, sun radiation, dampness, drafts, changes in barometric pressure, high altitude, carbon dioxide, carbon monoxide, air conditioning; other types of radiation like computer, microwave, X-ray, geopathic radiation, electrical and electromagnetic radiation, fluorescent lights, radiation from cellular and cordless telephones, and radiation from power lines are irritants. Vibrations from a washer and dryer, hair dryer, electric shaver, massager, motion vibrations from a moving automobile, motion sickness (car sickness, sea sickness), sickness while playing sports, roller coaster rides and/or horseback riding are mechanical irritants. Airplane sounds, traffic noises, loud music and voices in a particular pitch may also cause allergic reactions. All the above are known as physical allergens. Burns may also be included in this category.

It is not uncommon for children with autism to suffer from repeated canker sores. They suffer from sluggish digestion due to many food allergies, and food remains longer in the small bowel. According to Oriental medical principles, when food remains in the small bowel too long, the undigested food produces a large amount of heat. The heat escapes through the mouth causing the delicate mucous membrane of the mouth to blister and form canker sores.

One of the young patients, Alan, who came to our office, had a history of canker sores whenever he ate pizza for dinner. He turned out to be highly allergic to tomato sauce (spices and tomato). After the basics, he was treated for tomato mix and pepper mix. He has never been bothered by canker sores again.

Many symptoms of autism spectrum patients become exaggerated on cold, cloudy or rainy days. The patients could suffer from a severe allergy to carbon dioxide (their own breath), electrolytes, cold or a combination of all. Some people, especially people who suffer from mental imbalances, also react to moonlight or moon radiation.

Some autism spectrum patients experience fear and anxiety attacks when taking a hot shower. They are also allergic to humidity and can be successfully treated with NAET. A glass jar with a lid is filled half way with hot water will serve as the sample. A NAET practitioner administers the NAET treatment while the patient or surrogate holds the jar. In certain cases, salt is added to the hot water sample, creating salty and humid vapor (in order to treat someone who reacts to the atmosphere in coastal climates). Samples of very hot water used in treatment of mild to moderate types of burns have shown excellent results. Cold, high altitude, low altitude, wind, dampness, dryness, rain water, and other physical agents can be treated in a similar way.

Some patients react to heat or cold violently, suffering from extreme chills and shaking uncontrollably. They need to bundle up with three-four layers of clothing during a cold day or experience icy cold hands and feet even if they are clad in mittens and warm socks. These patients are simply allergic to cold and combinations with other substances. An allergy to cold makes the blood sticky and the circulation will be poor. The body will not be able to get rid of its toxins. Allergy to antioxidants like vitamin C, A, etc. makes the elimination of the toxins difficult.

If patients are allergic to iron, hormones, heat, etc., their reactions are just the opposite in hot weather. They feel very uneasy at high temperature. They may need treatments for vitamin C, iron, cold, hormones, and their own blood, alone or in combination. When they finish the treatment program, they are less prone to feeling cold or getting sick from changes in temperature.

GENETIC FACTORS

Bea, 38-years-old, had suffered from various allergies since she was an infant. When she was three-weeks-old, she broke out in a rash, which transformed into big heat boils. Her parents tried various medications in attempts to cure her including allopathy, homeopathy, and herbal medicines. Finally, herbal medicine brought the problem somewhat under control. Even with the herbal treatment, she still occasionally suffered from outbreaks of skin lesions. When she was ten-years-old, she developed severe attention deficit and hyperactive disorder. She also suffered from headaches, severe insomnia, depression, and mood swings.

After evaluation, she was found to be reacting to parasites. We learned that both her parents were in the Peace Corps before she was born. They were somehow infected with parasites and were seriously ill for months, but had no idea that their health problems were caused by the parasites until later. After she was treated successfully with NAET for parasites, Bea's health took a quantum leap. Her learning disability and attention deficit and hyperactive disorders improved greatly.

MOLDS AND FUNGI

Many autistic children suffer from yeast, candida, mold, and fungus overgrowth in the body. People with autism can suffer from severe allergy to sugar, starches, and carbohydrates. Consumption and poor digestion of sugar products create yeast, candida, etc. in the gut of the person.

Overgrowth of these will cause them to travel to other parts of the body. Molds and fungi belong to the same family and share the same energy fields. Reactions to these substances make people irritable, depressed, and they can suffer from a variety of mental imbalances, which can be easily mistaken for autism. When they get appropriate treatment to eliminate their yeast, candida, mold and fungi, they become symptom-free.

Allergies to toilet papers, toilet seat covers, etc., also cause yeast-like infections in some people. One of the patients reacted to everything she ate from her freezer. More investigation proved that she was allergic to the molds found in her freezer.

EMOTIONAL FACTORS

Emotions can affect children who become autistic later. Sudden fears, frightening sights, etc. can give sudden shock to the child's brain and cause autism-like symptoms later.

Steven was six years old when he was brought to us for treatment of autism. He had been a normal child until he was two when his parents noticed abnormal behaviors. He was diagnosed with autism spectrum disorders when he was three. In our evaluation it was suspected that his autism was due to an emotional fear that happened when he was about two years old. He did not have any allergy to foods, environmental factors or immunizations. His parents could not remember any event causing possible fear at that age. So he was treated for general energy balancing. He and his parents were sent home to do some deep thinking, since NST was focusing on an emotional fear. On the following day his parents returned amazed at the NAET test results. They had forgotten that Steven, in fact, had a dangerous fall at around two. He fell in the swimming pool, lost consciousness, spent 36 hours in the hospital and recovered from that episode completely. Time healed the wound and the parents forgot the incident. But the child's subconscious mind did not come to a settlement until we treated him for the fear from that fall with NAET. Steven became normal once again.

Autistic children should be checked for all possible emotional blockages before and after birth. Monica was eight years old when she was brought to our clinic. This beautiful girl was born autistic. She was nonverbal, non-communicable with no eye contact. Any little noise made her scream and hide under the table or behind a door. While she was being examined, a fire engine passed by my office and she was frightened beyond description. Through NTP (NAET Testing Procedures) we detected a fear that had affected her while she was in the womb at eight months. Questioning her mother Sonya, it was revealed that something horrible had happened while she was pregnant and expecting her. Sonya had gone to do some shopping at about 10 A.M. When she returned to her condominium she found many fire trucks and police cars blocking her entry to the condominium. Her condo had burned down completely as well as the neighbors' on both sides. The fire had started in her condo; she had left some food cooking on the stove and forgot to turn it off when she went to the market. She was so devastated about the whole thing that she became very sick and began having labor pains. She was admitted to the hospital immediately and stayed for a couple of weeks until Monica was born.

Sonya's story supported the result of NTP. I believed that the fetus absorbed the fear and became autistic when born. We treated Monica for this fear as a first treatment and she calmed down after the treatment for fear. She continued NAET treatments for 18 months. Now she is a normal, beautiful, 16-year-old girl attending a regular high school.

Much research is needed to understand the mechanism of NAET testing that is able to detect the energy imbalance at the emotional level and bring the individual back to health prior to the particular incident soon after the correction of the imbalance using NAET treatment technique.

3

AUTISM SCREENING MODALITIES

Autism is classified as one of the pervasive developmental disorders. Some doctors also use terms such as "emotionally disturbed" to describe people with autism. Because it varies widely in its severity and symptoms, autism may go unrecognized, especially in mildly affected individuals, or in those with multiple handicaps. Researchers and therapists have developed several sets of diagnostic criteria for autism. All currently available diagnostic methods are quite subjective and have lots of shortcomings. Since there is no way of avoiding subjectivity, diagnosis by experts is no better than diagnosis by the various checklists. since no perfect diagnostic tests are available to diagnose autism, we are forced to use whatever is available and make the best use of it.

Parents are usually the first to notice unusual behaviors in their children. In many cases, their baby seemed "different" from birth - being unresponsive to people and toys, or focusing intently on one item for long periods of time. The first signs of autism may also appear in children who had been developing normally; when an affectionate, babbling toddler suddenly becomes silent, withdrawn, violent, or self-abusive, something is wrong.

Even so, years may go by before the family seeks a diagnosis. Well-meaning friends and relatives sometimes help parents ignore the problems with reassurances that "Every child is different," or "Janie can talk, she just doesn't *want* to!" Unfortunately, this only delays getting appropriate assessment and treatment for the child.

As I stated earlier, to date, there are no medical tests like x-rays or blood tests that detect autism, and no two children with the disorder behave the same way. In addition, several conditions can cause symptoms that resemble those of autism. So parents and the child's pediatrician need to rule out other disorders including: hearing loss, speech problems, mental retardation, and neurological problems. Once these possibilities have been eliminated, a visit to a professional who specializes in autism is necessary. Such specialists include people with the professional titles of child psychiatrist, child psychologist, developmental pediatrician, or pediatric neurologist.

Autism specialists use a variety of methods to identify the disorder. Using a standardized rating scale, the specialist closely observes and evaluates the child's language and social behavior. A structured interview is also used to elicit information from parents about the child's behavior and early development. Reviewing family videotapes, photos, and baby albums may help parents recall when each behavior first occurred and when the child reached certain developmental milestones. The specialists may also test for certain genetic and neurological problems.

After assessing observations and test results, the specialist makes a diagnosis of autism only if there is clear evidence of:

- poor or limited social relationships
- underdeveloped communication skills
- repetitive behaviors, interests, and activities.

People with autism generally have some impairment within each category, although the severity of each symptom may vary.

The diagnostic criteria also require that these symptoms appear by age three.

Some of the commonly used evaluation methods to diagnose autism are: diagnostic checklists completed by the parents (parents can answer about their children's activities better since the parents spend major part of their time with their children), rating the questions asked in the interviews by professionals, direct observation (this may not produce best results since children tend to be very different on different days and in different settings and also depends on their diet prior to the observation) and capturing the child's activity on a video at different settings and times.

Since most autistic children suffer from various food and environmental sensitivities, they all should be screened by NST-NAET (Neuromuscular sensitivity testing). NST (described in Chapter 6) can detect allergens easily and painlessly in a short period of time. Then the items found positive by NST should be tested again in the laboratory blood analysis via RAST (Radioaalergosorbant test) for the presence of antibodies to the suspected food and environmental substances (IgE Specific antigen study). IgE specific antigen test is very efficient to detect allergies.

Some frequently used criteria include:
- ♦ Absence or impairment of imaginative and social play
- ♦ Impaired ability to make friends with peers
- ♦ Impaired ability to initiate or sustain a conversation with others
- ♦ Stereotyped, repetitive, or unusual use of language
- ♦ Restricted patterns of interests that are abnormal in intensity or focus
- ♦ Apparently inflexible adherence to specific routines or rituals
- ♦ Preoccupation with parts of objects

NAMBUDRIPAD'S TESTING PROCEDURES (NTP)

1.   History

A complete history of the patient is taken from a parent. NAET Allergy Symptom Rating form (ASR), NAET Allergy Grading Scale (AGS), NAET Autism Rating tool, Childhood Autism Rating Scale (CARS), E2 form from Autism Research Institute are given to the parent or guardian. From these various check lists, the type and degree of autism is identified. Parents or caretakers usually observe this and have accurate information.

2.   Physical Examination

Observation of the mental status, face, skin, eyes, color, posture, movements, gait, tongue, scars, wounds, marks, body secretions, etc.

3.   Vital Signs

Evaluation of blood pressure, pulse, skin temperature and - palpable energy blockages as pain or discomfort in the course of meridians, etc.

4.   Neuromuscular Sensitivity Testing (NST)

The pool of electromagnetic energy around an object or a person allows an energy exchange. The human field absorbs the energy from the nearby object and processes it through the network of nerve energy pathways. If the foreign energy field shares suitable charges with the human energy field, the human field absorbs the foreign energy for its advantage and becomes stronger. If the foreign energy field carries unsuitable charges, the human energy field causes repulsion from it. These types of reactions of the human energy field can be determined by measuring the neuromuscular sensitivity. This can be done by electromyography. Or it can be done easily by using a NAET procedure called NST. NST is somewhat similar to MRT technique from applied kinesiology with a few added steps to insure the precision of the testing procedure. NST is one of the main components of NAET testing procedures and can be used as a communication pathway between the body and brain. Through NST, the patient can be tested for various allergens. NST is used by comparing the strength of a predetermined test muscle in the presence and absence of a suspected allergen. If the particular muscle (test muscle also called "indicator muscle") weakens in the presence of an item, it signifies that the item is an allergen. If the muscle remains strong, the substance is not an allergen. More explanation on NST will be given in Chapter 6. Only a few allergens can be screened at one session since this type of testing causes muscle fatigue both in the tester and in the subject. An autistic child may be tested through a surrogate.

5. EMF Test (Electro Magnetic Field Test)

The electromagnetic component of the human energy field can be detected with simple NST. The electro- magnetic field or human vibrations of people can also be measured by using the sophisticated electronic equipment developed by Dr. Valerie Hunt, Malibu, California. Dr. Hunt, a retired UCLA physics professor, has proven her theory of the Science of Human Vibrations through 25 years of extensive research and clinical studies. Her book, "*Infinite Mind,*" explains it in detail.

6. Radio-AllergoSorbant Test (RAST)

The radio-allergosorbant test or RAST measures IgE antibodies in serum by radioimmunoassay and identifies specific allergens causing allergic reactions. This test reveals immediate response to an allergen. Delayed reactions are not recorded in this test.

Blood counts, chemistry, lipid panels, etc. should be checked for any possible abnormalities. Usually autistic children show low levels of sodium in their body, and the autistic trait of craving salt.

These are the major tests we use in our office prior to beginning treatments. There are various checklists developed by various psychologists available. All of them are focused on diagnosing autism. One can use only a limited number of evaluations on any one individual. Otherwise one would be spending the entire time on evaluation only not in treatments. It is for the practitioner to select the best tests suitable for the individual patient. I also strongly recommend to enroll the autistic child in various available therapies near you: ABA, physical therapy, occupational therapy, speech therapy, meditation, yoga, exercise program, day camps, etc. If possible, home schooling should be avoided. Enroll them in a school, initially probably your child may need a special school, but as soon as he/she can sit in the regular school, you should enroll him/her in the regular school. Children are fast learners. Children learn from children. Watching other normal children of similar age, they learn appropriate imitation, behavior, peer relationships and mannerism in a normal setting. Some of the children who had home schooling had the slowest recovery when compared to children attended special schools and regular schools.

4

IS IT TRULY AUTISM?

T he diagnostic process for autism must begin with a formal medical history. Most people are interested in understanding the differences and/or the similarities of the methods of diagnosis, the effectiveness and length of treatment between traditional Western medicine and Oriental medicine. Since the purpose of this book is to provide information about the new treatment method of NAET, more attention will be given to Oriental medicine and NAET.

The American Psychiatric Association periodically publishes an updated manual of diagnostic criteria for various mental conditions and behavioral abnormalities. The most recent edition, as of this writing is the Diagnostic and Statistical Manual 1V-TR (DSM 1V-TR). It includes guidelines for diagnosis of autism. DSM 1V is for experienced professionals and is not intended for self-diagnosis of autism or any other condition described in the manual.

WHAT ARE THE SIGNS OF AUTISM?

Professionals who diagnose autism use the diagnostic criteria set forth by the American Psychiatric Association (1994), in The Diagnostic and Statistical Manual of Mental Disorders, DSM-1V-TR released in 2000.

According to DSM-1V the most obvious signs associated with this disorder are inattentiveness (short attention span, failure to listen, failure to follow instructions, inability to finish projects and stay focused); severe language deficits, social isolation, uneven fine and gross motor skills, temper tantrums and insistence on sameness.

In addition to these problems, depending on the child's age and developmental stage, parents and teachers may see temper tantrums, frustration, anger, bossiness, difficulty in following rules, disorganization, social rejection, low-self esteem, poor academic achievement, and inadequate self-application.

There are many books written on the subject of autism and every book you read will give you the standard criteria or diagnostic guidelines to detect and diagnose autism. I am not going into details about diagnosing an autistic child or adult through standard criteria in this book. But I am going to spend some time explaining things that you absolutely need to understand to recognize this health disorder, so that you can get appropriate help.

THE BEST DIAGNOSTIC TOOL

A detailed clinical history is the best diagnostic tool for any medical condition.

It is extremely important for the patient or his/her parents or guardians to cooperate with the physician in giving all possible information about the child to the doctor in order to obtain the best results. It is my hope that this chapter will help bring about a clearer understanding between NAET specialists and their patients; because, in order to obtain the most satisfactory results, both parties must work together as a team.

The doctor should gather a detailed history of the child before formulating a diagnosis of autism. Your doctor's office may ask you to complete a relevant questionnaire during your first appointment. It is important to cooperate with the office staff and provide as accurate a history as possible.

THE AUTISTIC PATIENT-QUESTIONNAIRE

Prenatal History:

(Socio-economic factors, exposures to substance abuse, cadmium, lead, mercury, coffee, alcohol, chemical toxins, carbon monoxide poisoning, bacterial toxins, emotional traumas during fetal development), delivery, birth records including birth weight and APGAR scores.

GROWTH AND DEVELOPMENTAL HISTORY

Illness During Infancy

Colic ——

Constipation ——

Diarrhea ——

Feeding problem ——

Excessive vomiting ——

Excessive white coating on the tongue ——

Excessive crying ——

Poor sleep ——

Disturbed sleep ——

Frequent ear infection ——

Frequent fever ——

Immunizations ——

Response to immunizations ——

Common childhood diseases like measles, chicken pox, mumps, strep-throat, etc.——

Any other unusual events (fire in the house, accidents, earthquakes, etc.) ——

DEVELOPMENTAL MILESTONES

Age Of The Child

Walked alone ——

Talked ——

Toilet trained for bladder and bowel ——

Enrolled in school ——

Medical History:

Surgeries ——

Hospitalizations ——

Diseases ——

Allergies ——

Frequent colds ——

Fevers ——

Ear infections ——

Asthma ——

Hives ——

Bronchitis ——

Pneumonia ——

Seizures ——

Sinusitis ——

Headaches ——

Vomiting ——

Diarrhea ——

Current medication ——

Any reaction to medication ——

Antibiotics and drugs taken ——

Parasitic infestation ——

Visited other countries ——

Social History:

Learning: responsiveness to teaching methods, interaction between friends and teachers, interaction between family members, activities at school, ability to speak, ability to learn sign language if unable to speak (many autistic children seem to be deaf and dumb), phobias, problems with discipline, and language delays.

Behaviors: cooperative, uncooperative, disruptive and/or aggressive behaviors; overactive, restless, or very passive, inattentive, uncooperative with his/her peers and adults.

Habits: temper tantrums, excessively active, constantly moving in seat or room, low self esteem, short attention span, unusual fears.

Hobbies: collecting things, painting, coloring, singing, etc.

Family History:

The medical history of the immediate relatives, mother, father, and siblings should be noted. The same questions are asked about the patient's relatives: grandparents, aunts, uncles, and cousins. A tendency to get sick or have allergies is not always inherited directly from the parents. It may skip generations or manifest in nieces or nephews rather than in direct descendants.

Information should also be sought about alcoholism, drug abuse, mental disorders, and other health disorders. The careful NAET specialist will also determine whether or not diseases such as tuberculosis, cancer, diabetes, rheumatic or glandular disorders exist, or have ever occurred in the patient's family history. All of these facts help give the NAET specialist a more complete picture of the hereditary characteristics of the patient. A tendency is inherited. It may be manifested differently in different people. Unlike the tendency, an actual medical condition such as autism is not always inherited. Parents may have had cancer or rheumatism, but the child can manifest that allergic inheritance as autism.

Present History:

When the family history is complete, the practitioner will need to look into the history of the patient's chief complaint and its progression. Some typical preliminary questions include: "When did your child's first symptom occur?" Did you notice your child's problem when he/she was an infant or a child, or did you first notice the symptoms during adolescence, or fully grown? Did it occur after going through a certain procedure? For example, did it occur for the first time after a dental procedure like a root canal, the first antibiotic treatment or after installing a water filter? Did it occur after acquiring a water-bed, tricycle, or after a booster dose of immunization or vaccination? One of my patients reported that her son's autism began a few months after he received a booster dose of MMR.

Once a careful history is taken, the practitioner often discovers that the patient's first symptoms occurred in early childhood. He or she may have suffered from infantile eczema, or asthma, but never associated it with autism, which may not have appeared until a later age.

Next, the doctor will want to know the circumstances surrounding and immediately preceding the first symptoms. Typical questions will include: "Did you change the child's diet or put him/her on a special diet? Did he/she eat something that he/she hadn't eaten lately, (perhaps for two or three months)? Did you feed him/her one type of food repeatedly, every day for a few days? Did the symptoms follow a childhood illness, (whooping cough, measles, chicken pox, diphtheria, polio) or any immunization for such an illness? Did they follow some other illness such as influenza, pneumonia or a major operation? Did the problem begin after your vacation to an island, to another country, or after an insect bite? When did the first symptom appear?

Any one of these factors can be responsible for triggering a severe allergic manifestation or precipitate the first noticeable symptoms of an allergic condition. Therefore, it is very important to obtain full and accurate answers when taking the patient's medical history.

Other important questions relate to the frequency and occurrence of the attacks. Although foods may be a factor, if the symptoms occur only at specific times of the year, the trouble most likely is due to pollens. Often a patient is sensitive to certain foods but has a natural tolerance that prevents sickness until the pollen sensitivity adds sufficient allergens to throw the body into an imbalance. If symptoms occur only on specific days of the week, they are probably due to something contacted or eaten on that particular day.

The causes of autism in different patients can, at first, appear random. Regular attacks of mental irritability was caused in one patient after eating potato chips. The super heated fat in the potato chips caused a severe reaction in this child. Another child refused to eat anything but deep fried foods. Brain irritability in this patient caused depletion of fatty acids. He was highly allergic to all components of fat: animal fat, vegetable fat, fatty acids, and deep fried fatty finger foods, etc.). A child of eight suffered severe insomnia on Friday nights. The cause was traced to the Friday night's traditional pizza. A 29-year-old autistic man complained of a severe headache every Sunday morning. The cause was traced to eating a traditional Italian dish every Saturday night with his family. He was allergic to the tomato in the food. A young patient had an allergic attack of sneezing, runny nose, mental irritability, and headaches on Friday night. I traced the allergy to the chemical compounds in her coloring books.

The time of day when the attacks occur is also of importance in determining the cause of an allergic manifestation. If it always occurs before mealtime, hypoglycemia may be a possible cause. If it occurs after meals, an allergy to carbohydrates and starch complexes or something in the meal should be suspected. If it occurred regularly at night, it is quite likely that there is something in the bedroom that is aggravating the condition. It may be that the patient is sensitive to: feathers in the pillow or comforter, wood cabinets, marble floors, carpets, side tables, end tables, bed sheets, pillows, pillow cases, detergents used in washing clothes, indoor plants, shrubs, trees, or grasses outside the patient's window. One of my patients suffered from severe insomnia and irritability at night. After spending a few minutes in bed, he regularly got up agitated and uptight and would spent the rest of the night without sleep. He was found to be allergic to his blue colored silk bed sheet and pillow cases; he was found to be allergic to the color blue, which instead of calming him, made him very restless.

Many patients react violently to house dust, different types of furniture, polishes, house plants, tap water and purified water.

The doctor should ask the patient to make a daily log of all the foods he/she is eating. The ingredients in the food should be checked for possible allergens. Certain common allergens like corn products, MSG (monosodium glutamate or Accent), citric acid, etc., are used in food preparations.

Cornstarch is used as a binding ingredient in almost all vitamins and pills, including aspirin and Tylenol. Cornstarch is also seen in baking powder, baking soda, detergent, etc. Corn syrup is the natural sweetener in many of the products we ingest, including soft drinks. Corn silk is found in cosmetics and corn oil is used as a vegetable oil. For sensitive people this food adds another nightmare.

Other common ingredients in many preparations that autistic people may react severely to are various gums (acacia gum, xanthine gum, karaya gum, etc.). Numerous gums are used in candy bars, yogurt, cream cheese, soft drinks, soy sauce, barbecue sauce, fast food products, macaroni and cheese, etc.

Carob, a staple in many health food products, is another item that causes brain irritability among allergic people. Many health-conscious people are turning to natural food products in which carob is used as a chocolate and cocoa substitute. It is also used as a natural coloring or stiffening agent in soft drinks, cheeses, sauces, etc. We discovered that some of the causes of "holiday flu" and depression during holiday season are due to allergies to carob, chocolate, and turkey.

When assessing a child in whom autism is suspected, care must be taken not to misdiagnose him/her. Misdiagnosis of autism can probably hurt the child and the family's peace of mind for a long time

As I have stated earlier, in my opinion, the majority of people labeled as having autism are not suffering from autism. They may be suffering from simple undiagnosed allergies.

5

THE MISSING LINK

The word "kinesiology" refers to the science of movement. It was first proposed in 1964 by George Goodheart, a Detroit doctor of chiropractic. As a function of his practice, Dr. Goodheart learned a great deal about a patient's condition by using isolated movements of various muscles. Isolation techniques, a chiropractic procedure, made it possible to test the strength of an individual muscle or muscle group without the help of other muscles. Dr. Goodheart, with the help of a group of chiropractors, concluded after many experiments that structural imbalance causes disorganization of the entire body. This disorganization results in specific disorders of the glands, organs, and central nervous system. His findings were similar to what pioneer Chinese doctors had observed.

Kinesiology holds that when the body is disorganized, the structural balance or electrical force is not functioning normally. When that happens, the electrical energy life force doesn't flow freely through the nerve cells and causes energy blockages in the person. According to the Chinese, the free flow of energy is necessary for the normal functioning of the body. When your flow of energy gets blocked, you become ill. The energy and the messages travel from cell to cell in nanoseconds.

The messages both from and to the brain also pass through this energy channel.

Many years ago, pioneer Chinese doctors and philosophers studied these energy pathways and networks of the human body's energy system by observing living people and their normal and abnormal body functions. The Chinese learned to manipulate these energy pathways, or meridians, to the body's advantage. About 4,000 years ago, there was no scientific equipment available to feel or observe the presence of the energy flow and its pathways. Now, it is possible to study and trace the energy flow and pathways by using Kirlian photography and radioactive tracer isotopes. Although the existence of energy pathways in the human body has only been confirmed relatively recently, the Chinese doctors hypothesized and established their existence long ago.

Chinese medical theory points out that free-flow of Chi or energy through the meridians is necessary to keep the body in perfect balance. In the United States during the late 19th century, the founder of Chiropractic medicine, Daniel David Palmer, said, "Too much or too little energy is sickness." Even though it is believed that Palmer may have had no knowledge of Chinese medicine, his theory corresponded with the ancient Chinese theory of "free flowing energy."

Through Dr. Palmer, doctors of chiropractic learned about the importance of stabilizing energy and manipulating the spinal segments and nerve roots to keep them perfectly aligned, bringing the body to a balanced state. In the East, acupuncture developed based on the ancient Chinese theory. Eastern acupuncturists tried to bring balance by manipulating the energy meridians at various acupuncture points, inserting needles to remove blockages and reinstating the "free flow of Chi" along the energy pathways. East and West, unaware of each other's findings, worked in a similar manner toward the same goal: to balance the energy and to free sick people from their pain and illness.

Both groups realized that the overflow or underflow of energy, or in other words, too much or too little energy is the cause of an imbalance. When the flow is reinstated, the balance is restored.

NAET - THE MISSING LINK

A trained acupuncturist can differentiate between the overflow and underflow of Chi, and the affected meridians and organs. Balance is achieved faster when treatment is administered to strengthen the hypo-functioning organ, while draining the overflowing meridians and the organs. This is the practice of acupuncture. NTP and NAET are built on acupuncture theory, but have taken it one step further. Using the ideas from acupuncture theory, without necessarily using actual needle insertion, meridians can be unblocked, overflowing meridians can be drained and the excess energy can be rerouted through the empty meridians and associated organs. Thus the entire body reaches homeostasis. NAET is perhaps the missing link that various professionals have been searching for years to find.

When the body senses a danger or a threat from an allergen, sensory nerves carry the message to the brain and the brain in turn alerts the whole body about the imminent danger. Muscles contract to conserve energy, other defense forces like lymph, blood cells, etc., get ready to face the emergency. Spinal nerves also get tightened due to the contracted muscles. Vertebrae go into misalignment causing impingement at the affected vertebral level. Energy is blocked due to the impingement. So, a good chiropractic adjustment can remove the nerve impingement at the specific vertebral level and this can unblock the blocked energy pathway, freeing the energy to circulate again.

Herbs can cause similar healing. Electromagnetic forces of special herbs actually have the ability to enter selective energy pathways and push energy blockages out of the body to restore the energy balance. A well-trained herbalist can bring about results similar to that of a NAET specialist. Chiropractic, kinesiology, acupuncture, and herbology are blended together to create NAET.

Brain chemicals are not produced or distributed correctly in autistic patients. If given a chance, appropriate stimulation to the spinal nerves, the brain, and nervous system, can produce substances within the body and distribute them appropriately. These substances include: adrenaline, thyroxin, pituitropin, serotonin, dopamine, endorphin, dynorphin, enkephalin, interferon, cytokines, interleukin, leukotriene, prostaglandin, and other immune mediators to heal many problems. As long as the brain receives the right directions and commands, the brain has the ability to create appropriate remedial secretions that release to the target tissue and organs when needed, thus healing infections, allergies, imbalances, immune deficiency diseases, etc.,. This has been demonstrated repeatedly and proven in many cases when treated with NAET.

When body functions do not take place freely, the body begins to succumb to health problems: fatigue, headaches, sleep disturbances, irritability, forgetfulness, confusion, depression, craving, eating disorders, difficulty in thinking, poor concentration, phobias, crying spells, suicidal thoughts, burning sensations on the skin and on the limbs i.e. hands, feet, palms and soles, and feelings of loneliness even in crowds. Many of these symptoms are experienced by autistic patients.

If you fail to eliminate the blockage immediately, the adverse energy eventually takes over the body and causes problems at deeper levels. For example, headaches can turn into irritability, hyperactivity, and other brain disorders; neuropsychological complaints such as anger, irritability, confusion, and depression, etc., may turn the sufferer into a psychiatric case, possibly leading to institutionalization.

In our modern society, where color televisions are abundant, young mothers place infants in front of the television while they sit and watch television themselves or while doing chores. Infants get attracted by sudden changing colors and flashing on the screen, and stare at it in amazement while absorbing the radiation emitted by the television set. If the infant is allergic to radiation, and if the radiation affects his brain, he is going to be growing up with abnormalities in the brain function and can eventually suffer from ADD, ADHD, or autism.

The nervous system is without a doubt the most complex, widely investigated and least understood system in the body. Its structures and activities are interwoven with every aspect of our lives: physical, cultural, and intellectual. Investigators of many different disciplines, all holding their own methodologies, motivations, and persuasions, converge in the study of the nervous system. Depending on the context, there are many appropriate ways of embarking upon a study of the nervous system.

One of the primary functions of the human nervous system is gathering and processing information. Millions of minor adjustments are constantly being made automatically without our conscious knowledge or having to make a decision, as the total human being consciously senses and responds, according to the stimuli presented by the environment. For instance, when you are hot, you consciously move yourself away from the sun, or turn on the air conditioning. But the body is already making several hundred minor adjustments that trigger changes in the blood flow and the heart rate, expanding and contracting the blood vessels near the skin surfaces, activating the lymph glands, turning on the sweat glands, and so on without our knowing or thinking about it. These actions of the autonomic nervous system are preprogrammed into every cell of the body that responds to conscious activity. The autonomic responses are constantly readjusting to respond appropriately to the changing environment.

It is extremely important to recognize the body's attempts to maintain a homeostatic state (balance within the organism). The total balance takes place in various steps, utilizing assistance from a number of functional units. These functional units are large bodies of tissues composed of many microscopic cells, each having a specialized job in the body. These special tissues provide assistance in creating homeostasis at the lowest levels, within the individual's cells themselves.

The process through which homeostasis occurs is very complex, requiring considerable understanding of the biochemical and bioelectrical properties of the cells. Simplified, it can be said that all cells are surrounded by a plasma membrane similar to a microscopic plastic bag. The walls of this membrane are thick enough to contain the intracellular materials while maintaining the cell shape and size. It is also strong enough to protect the cells from invasion of the extracellular materials that surround each and every cell.

The ionic or magnetic properties of the atoms that make up the fluids inside the cell differ from the fluids of the surrounding cells. Because of the differences in ionic composition, there are differences in their electrical properties or charges. The difference in electrical energies can be measured in laboratory experiments on various kinds of tissues. In addition, it can assess the individual cell's responses to the electrical charges, which add up to millions of measurements per minute. Conversely, it is thin enough and permeable enough to allow the free flow of nutrients.

As a stimulus is applied at some point on the organism, it sets up a sequence of events which are eventually transmitted to the surfaces of excitable cells. The cells in turn redistribute the ions across the surface of the cell membrane by a process called osmosis. Osmosis is a transient, reversible, wave of change which affects the permeability of cell membranes, allowing fluids to both penetrate and flow out of the cell. The transfer of fluids temporarily changes the cell's shape, size, and function until it returns to its original or homeostatic state.

In all unicellular and some primitive multicellular forms of life, individual cells are capable of reacting to stimuli; whereas most complex life forms consist of a nervous system of specific cells which process and interpret stimuli. Thus, in the human body there are highly specialized receptor cells, which function to receive stimuli. These receptor cells work in harmony with neurons or nerve cells for the integration and conduction of information The effector cells (the contractile and glandular cells) mediate the action of the body's responses which start at the cellular level.

This is the foundational premise upon which the understanding of allergies is based; the neuromuscular sensitivity testing detects allergies and NAET eliminates allergies.

The ability of the central nervous system to react almost instantaneously to a stimulus such as the sensation of heat, cold, smell, etc., even on the most remote part of the extremities, is the result of the nervous system's interpretation and reaction to stimuli. The body is made up of trillions of individually well-equipped cells. Each cell has the memory to reproduce any number of chemicals and functions in the body. For some reason, in autistic patients, some of these cells remain dormant or have lost the memory to reproduce the neurochemicals or appropriate neurotransmitters. Due to the inactive chemical messengers, messages are not transmitted appropriately from neuron to neuron. Therefore, the nervous system of the autistic person does not work as smoothly as a normal person's nervous system.

If a stimulus is not short-circuited by nerve damage, blockage, or missed chemical response due to some defect in the neurotransmitters it reaches the brain where the message is accepted. Instantaneously the brain formulates a response and transmits it to all the receptors in the body. In turn, the receptors receive the message as either harmful or harmless. If the receptors receive the message as harmful, they repel it and transmit their response to the brain. If more stimuli with negative information reaches the brain, the brain accepts the rejection message from the majority of receptors; thus setting into motion evasive reactions. In the event that the body cannot effectively avoid or reject the stimulus, it will set up a reaction in an effort to cleanse itself of the stimulus. In an autistic person, incorrect or incomplete stimulus reaches the brain repeatedly and as a result inappropriate responses are ongoing.

Activities of the sympathetic system prepare the body for increased activities. The action of the sympathetic system is characterized by the formation of biochemicals such as noradrenaline and adrenaline along with some other basic enzymes, which prepare the body for reaction.

Chiropractors and acupuncturists stimulate the sympathetic nerve activity, by removing the nerve energy blockages, thus reinstating the nerve energy circulation in the body. These two groups of medical practitioners from East and West have learned to manipulate the sympathetic nerves to the patient's advantage, which in turn promotes healing power within the body, without the introduction of foreign chemicals/medications.

It is sufficient to say that even a very minor stimulus sensed by any receptor nerve cell located on the body, will set into motion the manufacturing process of hundreds of different kinds of chemicals; each assists the nerves in producing appropriate responses to the particular stimulus. Beyond this point, the nervous system becomes a matter of complicated medical study.

6

NAET TESTING PROCEDURES

When a person comes close to the energy field of a substance, if that energy field happened to be incompatible to the individual, then a repulsion of the two energy fields take place. The substance that is capable of producing the repulsion between the energy fields of the individual and the substance itself is considered an allergen to the particular individual. We frequently go near allergens and interact with their energies without recognizing this repulsive action, whether from foods, drinks, chemicals, environmental substances, animals or other humans. This causes energy disturbances in the meridians; thereby causing imbalances in the body. The imbalances cause illnesses, which create disorganization in body functions. The disorganization of the body and its functions involve the vital organs, their associated muscle groups, and nerve roots which can give rise to brain disorders. To prevent the allergen from causing further disarray after producing the initial blockage, the brain sends messages to every cell of the body to reject the presence of the allergen. This rejection will appear as repulsion, and the repulsion will produce different symptoms related to the affected organs.

Your body has an amazing way of telling you when you are in trouble. If you went for help at the earliest hint of need, you would save yourself from unnecessary pain and agony. As a matter of habit, you often have to be hurting severely before you seek help. This applies to allergies, too. If you have a way to identify the allergens that can possibly cause reactions on your body way before you get exposed to them, you can simply avoid them and won't have to suffer the consequences. Now you have a way to do just that through NAET testing procedures (NAET Testing procedures are described in the following pages).

When some people go near allergens, they receive various clues from the brain, such as: an itchy throat, watery eyes, sneezing attacks, coughing spells, unexplained pain anywhere in the body, yawning, sudden tiredness, etc. You can demonstrate these changes by testing the strength of any part of the body in the presence and absence of the allergen. A strong muscle of the arm, hand or leg can be used for this test. Test a strong muscle for its strength away from the allergen, and then test it again in the presence of the allergen and compare the strength. The muscle will stay strong without any allergen near the body, but will weaken in the presence of an allergen. This response of the muscle can be used to your advantage to demonstrate the presence of an allergen near you.

NEURO MUSCULAR SENSITIVITY TESTING OF NAMBUDRIPAD'S ALLERGY ELIMINATION TECHNIQUES (NST-NAET ®)

NST is one of the tools used by NAET® specialists to test imbalances and allergies in the body. The same muscle response testing can also be used to detect various allergens that cause imbalances in the body.

Neuromuscular sensitivity testing can be performed in the following ways (Illustrations of different types of NST can be seen on the following pages).

1. Standard NST can be done in standing, sitting or lying positions. You need two people to do this test: the person, who is testing, or the "tester," and the subject, the person being tested.

2. The "Oval Ring Test" can be used in testing yourself, and on a very strong person with a strong arm.

3. Surrogate testing can be used to test an infant, invalid person, extremely strong or very weak person, or an animal. The surrogate's muscle is tested by the tester, and the subject maintains skin-to-skin contact with the surrogate while being tested. The surrogate does not get affected by the testing. NAET® treatments can also be administered through the surrogate very effectively without causing any interference with the surrogate's energy.

NEURO MUSCULAR SENSITIVITY TESTING (NST)

Two people are required to perform standard neuromuscular sensitivity testing: the tester, and the subject. The subject can be tested lying down, standing, or sitting. The lying-down position is the most convenient for both tester and subject; it also achieves more accurate results.

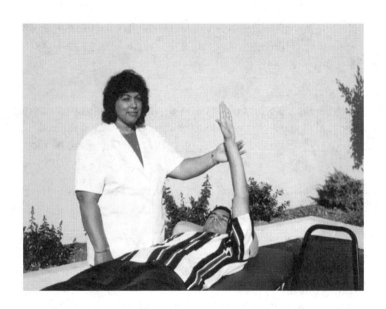

FIGURE 1
NST WITHOUT ALLERGEN

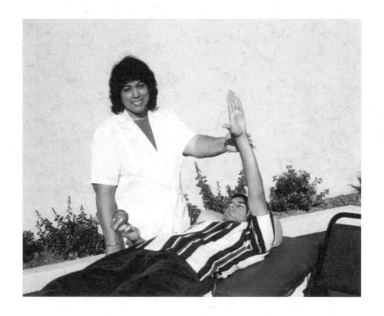

Figure   2

TESTING WITH ALLERGEN

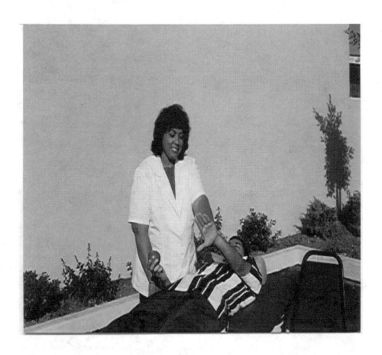

Figure   3
NST WITH ALLERGEN

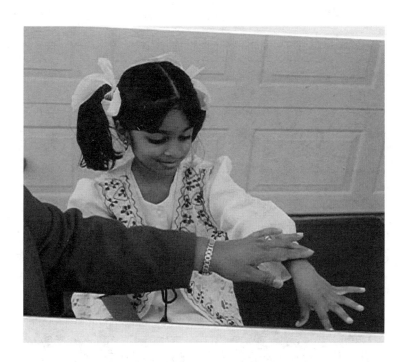

FIGURE 4
NST IN STANDING POSITION

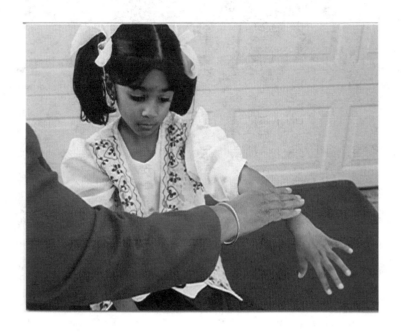

FIGURE 5
NST IN SITTING POSITION

Step 1:   The subject lies on a firm surface with the left arm raised 45-90 degrees to the body with the palm facing outward and the thumb pointing toward the big toe.

Step 2: The tester stands on the subject's (right) side. The subject's right arm is kept to his/her side with the palm either kept open to the air, or in a loose fist. The fingers should not touch any material, fabric or any part of the table the arm is resting on because this can give wrong test results. The tester's left palm is contacting the subject's left wrist (Figure 6-1).

Step 3: It is essential to test a strong predetermined muscle (PDM) to get accurate results. The tester using the left arm tries to push the raised arm toward the subject's left big toe. The subject resists the push. The arm, or pre-determined indicator muscle, remains strong if the subject is well balanced at the time of testing. If the muscle or raised arm is weak and gives way under pressure without the presence of an allergen, either the subject is not balanced, or the tester is performing the test improperly; for example, the tester might be trying to overpower the subject. The subject does not need to gather up strength from other muscles in the body to resist the tester. Only 5 to 10 pounds of pressure needs to be applied for three to five seconds. If the muscle shows weakness, the tester will be able to judge the difference with only that small amount of pressure.

Step 4: This step is used if the patient is found to be out of balance as indicated by the PDM presenting weak without the presence of an allergen. The tester then uses the balancing points by placing the fingertips of right hand at Point 1. The left hand is placed on Point 2 (see below and figure 6-6). The tester massages these two points gently clockwise with the fingertips about 20-30 seconds, and then repeats steps 2 and 3. If the PDM tests strong, continue on to step 5.

Point 1:
Name of the point: Sea of Energy

Location: Two finger-breadths below the navel, on the midline. According to Oriental medical theory, this is where the energy of the body is stored in abundance. When the body senses any danger around its energy field or when the body experiences energy disturbances, the energy supply is cut short and stored here. If you massage clockwise on that energy reservoir point, the energy will come out of this storage and travel to the part of the body where it is needed.

Point 2:

Name of the point: Dominating Energy

Location: In the center of the chest on the midline of the body, level with the fourth intercostal space. This is the energy dispenser unit. When the energy rises from the Sea of Energy, it goes straight to the Dominating Energy point. This is the point that controls and regulates the energy circulation or Chi, in the body. From here, the energy is dispersed to different meridians, organs, tissues and cells as needed to help remove the energy disturbances. It does this by forcing energy circulation from inside out. Continue this procedure for 30 seconds to one minute and retest the NST. If the NST is found weak repeat the procedure until it gets strong. Check NST every 30 seconds.

Step 5: If the PDM remains strong when tested - a sign that the subject is balanced - then the tester should put the suspected allergen into the palm of the subject's resting hand. When the subject's fingertips touch the allergen, the sensory receptors sense the allergen's charges and relay the message to the brain. If it is an

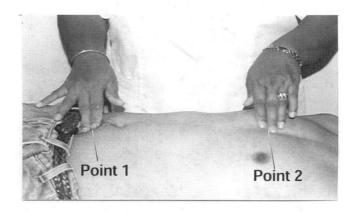

Point 1   Point 2

FIGURE 6
INITIAL BALANCING

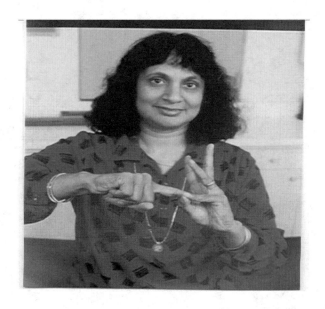

FIGURE 7
"O" Ring Testing

incompatible charge, the strong PDM will go weak. If the charges are compatible to the body, the indicator muscle will remain strong. This way, you can test any number of items to determine the compatible and incompatible charges.

Much practice is needed to test and sense the differences properly. If you can't test properly or effectively the first few times, don't get discouraged. Practice makes perfect.

"OVAL RING TEST" OR "O RING TEST"

The "Oval Ring Test" or "O Ring Test" can be used in self-testing. This can also be used to test a subject, if the subject is very strong physically with a strong arm and the tester is a physically weak person. (See figure 6-7)

Step 1: The tester makes an "O" shape by opposing the little finger and thumb on the same hand (finger pad to finger pad). Then, with the index finger of the other hand he/she tries to separate the "O" ring against pressure. If the ring separates easily, the tester needs to be balanced as described above.

Step 2: If the "O" ring remains inseparable and strong, hold an allergen in the other hand, by the fingertips, and perform step 1 again. If the "O" ring separates easily, the person is allergic to the substance in the hand. If the "O" ring remains strong, the substance is not an allergen.

NST is one of the most reliable methods of allergy tests, and it is fairly easy to learn and practice in every day life. It cuts out expensive laboratory work.

After considerable practice, some people are able to test very efficiently using these methods. It is very important for allergic people to learn some form of self-testing technique to screen out contact with possible allergens to prevent allergic reactions in

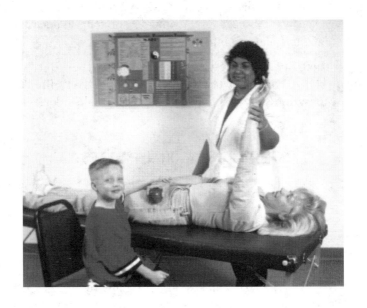

FIGURE 8
TESTING A TODDLER
THROUGH A SURROGATE

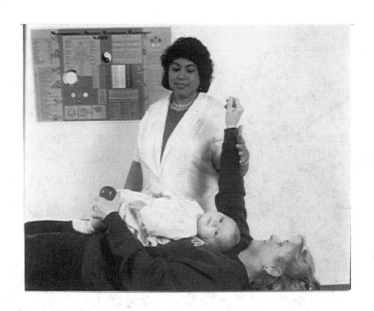

FIGURE 9
TESTING AN INFANT
THROUGH A SURROGATE

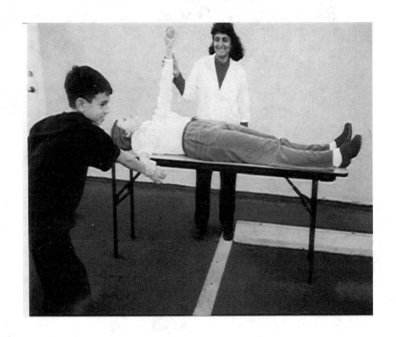

FIGURE 10
TESTING A HYPERACTIVE CHILD

order to have freedom to live in this chemically polluted world. After receiving the basic 30-40 treatments from a NAET practitioner, a person can test and avoid unexpected allergens. Hundreds of new allergens are thrown into the world daily by people who do not understand the predicament of allergic people. If you or your child want to live in this world looking and feeling normal among normal people, and side by side with the allergens, you need to learn how to test on your own. It is not practical for people to treat thousands of allergens from their surroundings or go to a NAET practitioner every day. If you learn to detect your allergies on your own after treating for NAET basics, you and your child can live without many health problems.

A TIP TO MASTER SELF-TESTING

Find two items, one that you are allergic to and another that you are not, for example an apple and a banana.

You are allergic to the apple and not allergic to the banana. Hold the apple in the right hand and do the "Oval Ring Test" as shown in the figure 6-7. The ring easily breaks. The first few times if it didn't break, make it happen intentionally. Now hold the banana and do the same test. This time the ring doesn't break. Put the banana down; rub your hands together for 30 seconds. Take the apple and repeat the testing. Practice this until you can sense the difference. When you can feel the difference between these two items you can test anything around you.

SURROGATE TESTING

This method can be very useful to test and determine the allergies of an infant, a child, a hyperactive child, an autistic child, disabled person, an unconscious person, an extremely strong, and a very weak person. You can also use this method to test an animal, plant, and a tree.

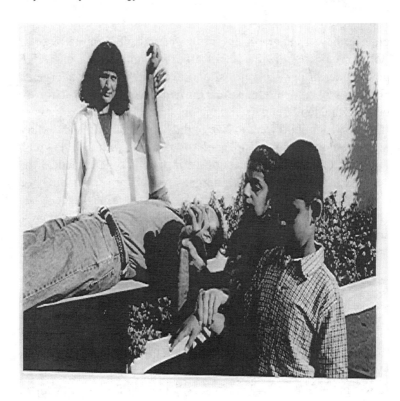

FIGURE 11
TESTING THROUGH AN EXTENDED SURROGATE

TESTING THROUGH AN EXTENDED SURROGATE

Extended surrogate testing is used when the patient is uncooperative, i.e. hyperactive, autistic, or frightened. Three people are needed for this test as shown in Figure 6-11. NAET treatments can be administered through the extended surrogate very effectively without causing any interference to the surrogate's energy.

The surrogate's muscle is tested by the tester. It is very important to remember to maintain skin-to-skin contact between the surrogate and the subject during the procedure. If you do not, then the surrogate will receive the results of testing and treatment.

The testing or treatment does not affect the surrogate as long as the subject maintains uninterrupted skin-to-skin contact with the surrogate.

NST can be used to test any substance for allergies. Even human beings can be tested for each other in this manner. When allergic to another human (father, mother, son, daughter, grandfather, grandmother, spouse, caretaker, baby sitter, etc.) you or your child could experience similar symptoms just as you would with foods, chemicals, or materials.

ABOUT PERSON-TO-PERSON ALLERGIES

If people are allergic to each other, the allergy can affect a person in various ways: If the father and/or mother is allergic to the child, or child allergic to a parent or parents, the child can get sick or remain sick indefinitely. The same things can happen to the parents. If the husband is allergic to the wife or wife towards the husband, they might fight all the time and/or their health can be affected. The same things can happen among other family members. It is important to test family members and other immediate associates with your child for possible allergy, and if found, they should be treated for each other.

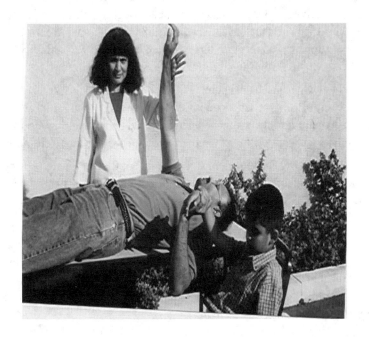

FIGURE   12

TESTING PERSON-TO-PERSON ALLERGY

TESTING PERSON-TO-PERSON ALLERGIES

The subject lies down and touches the other person he or she wants tested (Figure 6-12). The tester pushes the arm of the subject in steps 2 and 3 above. If the subject is allergic to the second person, the indicator muscle goes weak. If the subject is not allergic, the indicator muscle remains strong. This is done through a surrogate in autistic children. Sometimes, one needs to test an autistic or hyperactive child through an extended surrogate because the child may be violent or too strong for one surrogate to handle.

I strongly feel that NST for allergies should be taught in every school, every hospital, in all medical offices, and in every establishment. Everyone should learn to test and detect their allergies even if the treatment is not available. If you know your allergies, you can avoid many of them.

Let's look at the history of six -year-old David who suffered from severe autism for four years. His mother Diane brought David to the office regularly for treatments. Before the treatment, he was unable to hold any food down. He threw up every meal whether it was water or milk. He suffered from severe constipation, insomnia, irritability, colic pains and severe crying spells. He could not talk or communicate in words about his discomfort. Diane spent extra time in the office to learn about autism and the NAET connection. She also took special interest in the series of patient education seminars given in our office to the new patients. Through the patient education seminars she learned ways to detect David's untreated allergens before he was exposed to them. This made their lives easier.

She and her husband tested every food before they bought it from the store. Whenever they found an allergen, they avoided it until they brought the child to be treated to it with NAET. This helped David immensely. He stopped vomiting after each meal, skin rashes and hives began to diminish with each treatment, and he did not have many temper tantrums after this. He slept well without nightmares and crying spells.

Soon after David received about 15-20 treatments, his disposition changed. He started talking, and became friendlier; he was admitted to regular school. His mother became a teacher's assistant in his class so that she could keep close watch on him. His parents took special care to feed him allergy-tested or non-allergic food items so that he could continue normal activities. David responded well to the treatment faster than any other autistic child I had treated, and he was able to have a normal school life. He is a healthy, intelligent 15-year-old now.

As mentioned earlier, muscle response testing is one of the tools used by kinesiologists. Practiced in this country since 1964, it was originated by Dr. George Goodheart and his associates. The late Dr. John F. Thie advocated this method through the "Touch for Health" Foundation in Malibu, California. For more information and books available on the subject; interested readers can write to "Touch For Health" Foundation.

Just by knowing NST and testing procedures David's mother could prevent unwanted visits to the doctor's office. Most allergy related autism could be controlled if we can teach these simple testing skills to all the parents of autistic children, special education teachers, and caretakers, as well as encourage them to use non-allergic products in the house, schools, and work-place.

The theory of energy blockages and diseases comes from Oriental medicine. Oriental medicine also teaches that, if given a chance, with a little support, the body will heal itself.

7

SYMPTOMS OF MERIDIANS

T he human body is made up of bones, flesh, nerves and blood vessels, which can only function in the presence of vital energy. Like electricity, vital energy is not visible to the human eye.

No one knows how the vital energy gets into the body or how, when or where it goes when it leaves. It is true, however, that without it, none of the body functions can take place. When the human body is alive, vital energy flows freely through the energy pathways. Uninterrupted circulation of the vital energy flowing through the energy pathways is necessary to keep the person alive. This circulation of energy makes all the body functions possible. The circulation of the vital energy makes the blood travel through the blood vessels, helping to distribute appropriate nutrients to various parts of the body for its growth, development, functions, and for repair of wear and tear.

NAET has its origin in Oriental medicine. But if one explores most Oriental medical books–acupuncture textbooks, one may not find the NAET interpretation of health problems that I write in my books, because NAET is my sole development after observing my own reactions, my family's and patients' over the past two decades. Recently, however, Information about the effectiveness of NAET has been given credit in a number of books, but the reader will find correct information of NAET interpretation of Oriental medical principles only in my books.

In this book, information about acupuncture meridians are kept to a minimum, enough to educate the reader about some traditional functions and dysfunctions of the meridians in the presence of energy disturbances. Some of this information is also available in acupuncture textbooks that one may find in libraries. It is a good idea to have some understanding of Oriental medicine and the meridians when undergoing NAET treatments although it is not mandatory. To learn more about acupuncture meridians and mind-body connections, please read Chapter 10 in my book, *Say Good-bye to Illness.*

NAET utilizes a variety of standard medical procedures to diagnose and then treat allergies and allergy-related health conditions. These include: standard medical diagnostic procedures and standard allergy testing procedures (read Chapter 3). After detecting allergies, NAET uses standard chiropractic and acupuncture/acupressure treatments to eliminate them. Various studies have proven that NAET is capable of erasing the previously encoded incorrect message about an allergen and replacing it with a harmless or useful message by reprogramming the brain (Please read the Journal of NAET Energetics and Complementary Medicine,

Vol 1 and 2, 2005). This is accomplished by bringing the body into a state of "homeostasis" using various NAET energy balancing techniques.

Chiropractic theory postulates that a pinching of the spinal nerve root(s) may cause nerve energy disturbance in the energy pathways causing poor nerve energy supply to target organs. When the particular nerve fails to supply adequate amounts of energy to the organs and tissues, normal functions and appropriate enzymatic functions do not take place. The affected organs and tissues then begin to manifest impaired functions in digestion, absorption, assimilation and elimination. An allergy can also cause impaired functions of the organs and tissues themselves. In chiropractic theory, an allergy can be seen as a result of a pinched nerve. Impaired functions of the organs and tissues will improve when the pinching of the spinal nerves is removed and energy circulation is restored through chiropractic adjustments. But the adjustments have to be applied on a regular basis. Otherwise the misallignment could return.

I observed this phenomena on my regular chiropractic patients for a long time. I did not have an explanation for the need for "the twice a week" regular chiropractic treatment to keep the body in alignment. Then I combined NAET with regular chiropractic treatment. When these patients began desensitization for the NAET basic essential nutrients (NAET Basic allergens) through NAET, we noticed that they were holding adjustments for longer times. By the time they completed desensitization on 25 to 30 NAET Basic allergen, most of these patients responded very well healthwise. Their pains and other symptoms reduced greatly or eliminated completely. They digested their meals better. Sleep improved. Overall energy increased many fold. Their quality of life improved. They maintained their spinal alignments without losing them so they did not need frequent chiropractic adjustments as before. The observation of these patients invoked enough interest to study the benefits of NAET on a larger group and we received similar results. From this observation I concluded that allergens are the cause of spinal misalignments, pinched nerves and various other health disorders we see in people today.

Oriental medicine explains the same theory from a different perspective. In Oriental medicine, the balance of Yin and Yang represents the perfect balance of energies (the state of homeostasis). Any interference in the energy flow or an energy disturbance can cause an imbalance in the Yin-Yang state and an imbalance in "homeostasis." Any substance that is capable of creating an energy disturbance in one's body is called an allergen.

According to NAET theory, when a substance is brought into the electromagnetic field of a person, an attraction or repulsion takes place between the energy of the person and the substance.

ATTRACTION

If two energies are attracted to each other, both energies benefit each other. The person can benefit from association with the substance. The energy of the substance will combine with the energy of the person and enhance functional ability. For example: After taking an antibiotic, the bacterial infection is diminished. Here the energy of the antibiotic joins forces with the energy of the body and helps to eliminate the bacteria. Another example is taking vitamin supplements (if one is not allergic to them) and the gaining of energy and vitality.

REPULSION

If two energies repel each other, they are not good for each other. The person can experience the repulsion of his/her energy from the other as a pain or discomfort in the body. The energy of the person will cause energy blockages in his/her energy meridians to prevent invasion of the adverse energy into his/her energy field. For example: After taking a repelling antibiotic, not only does the bacterial infection not get better but the person might break out in a rash all over the body causing fever, nausea, excessive perspiration, light-headedness, etc. Another example is taking a repelling vitamin supplement one night and waking up with multiple joint pains and general body-ache the next morning. If repulsion takes place between two energies, then the substance that is capable of producing the repulsion in a living person is considered an allergen. When the allergen produces a repulsion of energy in the electromagnetic field, certain energy disturbance takes place in the body. The energy disturbance caused from the repulsion of the substance is capable of producing various unpleasant or adverse reactions. These reactions are considered "allergic reactions."

IMMUNOGLOBULINS

In certain instances, the body also produces many defensive forces like "histamine, immunoglobulins, etc." to help the body overcome the unpleasant reactions from the interaction with the allergen. The most common immunoglobulin produced during a reaction is called IgE (immunoglobulin E). These reactions are called IgE-mediated reactions.

An allergy means an altered reactivity. Reactions and after-effects can be measured using various standard medical diagnostic tests. Energy medicine has also developed various devices to measure the reactions. Oriental medicine has used "Medical I Ching" since 3,322 BC. Another simple way to test one's body is through simple, kinesiological neuromuscular sensitivity testing (NST) procedures (Chapter 6). It is an easy procedure for a person to evaluate his/her progress.

Study of the acupuncture meridians is helpful to understand NST and how it works. If one learns to identify abnormal symptoms connected with acupuncture meridians, detection of the causative agents (allergens) will be easier. The pathological functions of the twelve major acupuncture meridians follow:

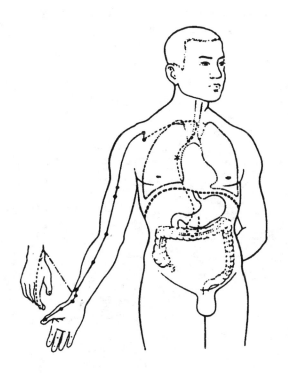

FIGURE 7-1

THE LUNG MERIDIAN (LU)

THE LUNG MERIDIAN (LU)

Energy disturbance in the lung meridian affecting physical and physiological levels can give rise to the following symptoms

Asthma between 3-5 a.m.
Atopic dermatitis
Bronchiectasis
Bronchitis
Burning in the eyes, & nostrils
Cardiac asthma
Chest congestion & cough
Coughing up blood
Cradle cap
Dry mouth, skin, throat
Emaciated look
Emphysema
Fever with chills
Frequent flu-like symptoms
General body ache with burning sensation
Generalized hives
Hair loss
Hair thinning
Hay-fever
Headache between eyes
Inability to sleep after 3 a.m.
Infantile eczema
Infection in the respiratory tract
Itching of the body, scalp, nose
Lack of desire to talk
Lack or excessive of perspiration
Laryngitis and pharyngitis
Low voice
Moles
Morning fatigue
Mucus in the throat
Nasal congestion or runny nose

Night sweats
Nose bleed
Pain between third and fourth thoracic vertebrae
Pain in the chest and intercostal muscles
Pain in the eyes
Pain in the first interphalangeal joint and thumb
Pain in the upper arms and back
Pain in the upper first and second cuspids (tooth)
Pleurisy
Pneumonia
Poor growth of nails and hair
Postnasal drip
Red cheeks and eyes
Restlessness between 3 to 5 a.m.
Scaly and rough skin
Sinus headaches and infection
Skin rashes
Skin tags
Sneezing
Sore throat
Stuffy nose
Swollen cervical glands
Swollen throat
Tenosynovitis
Thick yellow discharge in case of bacterial infection
Thin or thick white discharge in case of viral infection

Energy disturbance in the lung meridian affecting the cellular level. When one fails to cry, when one feels deep sorrow, sadness will settle in the lungs and eventually cause various lung disorders

Apologizing

Comparing self with others

Contempt

Dejection

Depression

Despair

False pride

Grief or sadness.

Highly sensitive emotionally

Hopelessness

Intolerance

Likes to humiliate others

Loneliness

Low self-esteem

Meanness

Melancholy

Over demanding

Over sympathy

Prejudice

Seeking approval from others

Self pity

Weeping Frequently

Essential Nutrients to Strengthen the Lung Meridian

Clear water

Proteins

Vitamin A

Vitamin C

Bioflavonoid

Cinnamon

Essential fatty acids

Onions

Garlic

B-vitamins (especially B_2)

Citrus fruits

Green peppers

Black peppers

Rice

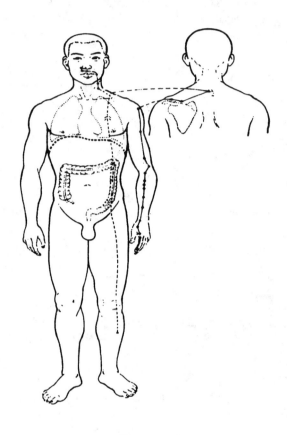

FIGURE 7- 2

THE LARGE INTESTINE MERIDIAN (LI)

THE LARGE INTESTINE MERIDIAN (LI)

Energy disturbance in the large intestine meridian affecting physical and physiological levels can give rise to the following symptoms

Abdominal pain
Acne on the face, sides of
   the mouth and nose
Asthma after 5 a.m.
Arthritis of the shoulder
   joint
Arthritis of the knee joint
Arthritis of the index
   finger
Arthritis of the wrist joint
Arthritis of the lateral part
   of the elbow and hip
Bad breath
Blisters in the lower gum
Bursitis
Dermatitis
Dry mouth and thirst
Eczema
Fatigue
Feeling better after a
   bowel movement
Feeling tired after a bowel
   movement
Flatulence
Inflammation of lower
   gum

Intestinal colic
Itching of the body
Loose stools or constipation
Lower backache
Headaches
Muscle spasms and pain of
lateral aspect of thigh, knee
   and below knee.
Motor impairment of the
fingers
 Pain in the knee
Pain in the shoulder,
   shoulder blade and back of
   the neck
Pain and swelling of the
   index finger
Pain in the heel
Sciatic pain
Swollen cervical glands
Skin rashes
Skin tags
Sinusitis
Tenosynovitis
Tennis elbow
Toothache
Warts on the skin.

Energy disturbance in the large intestine meridian affecting the cellular level can cause the following

Guilt

Confusion

Brain fog

Bad dreams

 dwelling on past memory

Crying spells

Defensiveness

Inability to recall dreams

 Nightmares

 Nostalgia

Rolling restlessly in sleep

Seeking sympathy

Talking in the sleep and Weeping

Essential Nutrients to Strengthen the Large Intestine Meridian

Vitamins A, D, E, C, B, especially B_1, wheat, wheat bran, oat bran, yogurt, and roughage.

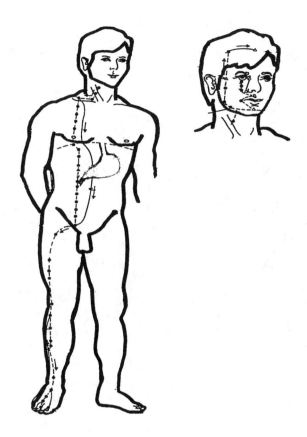

FIGURE 7-3

STOMACH MERIDIAN (ST)

THE STOMACH MERIDIAN (ST)

Energy disturbance in the stomach meridian affecting physical and physiological levels can give rise to the following symptoms

Abdominal Pains & distention
Acid reflux disorders
Acne on the face and neck
ADD & ADHD
Anorexia
Autism
Bad breath
Black/ blue marks on the
  leg below the knee
Bipolar disorders
Blemishes
Bulimia
Chest muscle pain
Coated tongue
Coldness in the lower limbs
Cold sores in the mouth
Delirium
Depression
Dry nostrils
Dyslexia
Excessive hunger
Facial paralysis
Fever blisters
Fibromyalgia
Flushed face
Frontal headache
Herpes

Heat boils (painful acne) in
the upper front of the body
Hiatal hernia
High fever
Learning disability
Insomnia due to nervousness
Itching on the skin & rashes
Migraine headaches
Manic depressive disorders
Nasal polyps
Nausea
Nosebleed
Pain on the upper jaws
Pain in the mid-back
Pain in the eye
Seizures
Sensitivity to cold
Sore throat
Sores on the gums & tongue
Sweating
Swelling on the neck
Temporomandibular joint
  problem
Unable to relax the mind
Upper gum diseases
Vomiting

Energy disturbance in the stomach meridian affecting the cellular level can cause the following

Disgust
Bitterness
Aggressive behaviors

Attention deficit disorders
Butterfly sensation in the
stomach

Essential Nutrients to Strengthen the Stomach Meridian

B complex vitamins especially B_{12}, B_6, B_3 and folic acid.

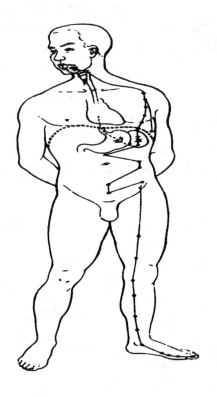

FIGURE 7-4

THE SPLEEN MERIDIAN (SP)

THE SPLEEN MERIDIAN (SP)

Energy disturbance in the spleen meridian affecting physical and physiological levels can give rise to the following symptoms

Abnormal smell
Abnormal taste
Abnormal uterine bleeding
Absence of menstruation
Alzheimer's disease
Autism
Bitter taste in the mouth
Bleeding from the mucous
  membrane
Bleeding under the skin
Bruises under the skin
Carpal tunnel syndrome
Chronic gastroenteritis
Cold sores on the lips
Coldness of the legs
Cramps after the first day of
  menses
Depression
Diabetes
Dizzy spells
Dreams that make you tired
Emaciated muscles
Failing memory
Fatigue in general
Fatigue of the mind
Fatigued limbs
Feverishness
Fibromyalgia
Fingers and hands-numbness
Fluttering of the eyelids
Frequent
Generalized edema
Hard lumps in the abdomen
Hemophilia

Hemorrhoids
Hyperglycemia
Hypertension
Hypoglycemia
Inability to make decisions
Incontinence of urine or stool
Indigestion
Infertility
Insomnia: usually unable to fall
asleep
Intractable pain anywhere in the
body
Intuitive and prophetic behaviors
Irregular periods
Lack of enthusiasm
Lack of interest in anything
Lethargy
Light-headedness
Loose stools
Nausea
Obesity
Pain and stiffness of the fingers
Pain in the great toes
Pallor
Pedal edema
Pencil-like thin stools with
undigested food particles
Poor memory
Prolapse of the bladder
Prolapse of the uterus
Purpura
Reduced appetite
Sand-like feeling in the eyes
Scanty menstrual flow

Sensation of heaviness in the
   body and head
Sleep during the day
Slowing of the mind
Sluggishness
Schizophrenia
Stiffness of the tongue
Sugar craving
Swelling anywhere in the body
Swellings or pain with swelling
   of the toes and feet

Swollen eyelids
Swollen lips
Tingling or abnormal sensation
   in the tip of the fingers and
   palms
Varicose veins
Vomiting
Watery eyes

Energy disturbance in the spleen meridian affecting the cellular level can cause the following

Anxiety
Concern
Does not like crowds
Easily hurt
Gives more importance to self
Hopelessness
Irritable
Keeps feelings inside
Lack of confidence
Likes loneliness
Likes to be praised
Likes to take revenge

Lives through others
Low self esteem
Needs constant encoragement
Obsessive compulsive
   behavior
Over sympathetic to others
Unable to make decisions
Restrained
Shy/timid
Talks to self
Worry

Essential Nutrients to Strengthen the Spleen Meridian

Vitamin A, vitamin C, calcium, chromium, protein, berries, asparagas, bioflavonoids, rutin, hesparin, hawthorn berries, oranges, root vegetables, and sugar.

THE HEART MERIDIAN (HT)

Energy disturbance in the heart meridian affecting the Physical and pysiological level can cause the following

Angina-like pains
Chest pains
Discomfort when reclining
Dizziness
Dry throat
Excessive perspiration
Feverishness
Headache
Heart palpitation
Insomnia—unable to fall asleep
When awakened in the middle
   of sleep

Heaviness in the chest
Hot palms and soles
Irritability
Mental disorders
Nervousness
Pain along the left arm
Pain along the scapula
Pain and fullness in the chest
Pain in the eye
Poor circulation
Shortness of breath
Shoulder pains

Energy disturbance in the heart meridian affecting the cellular level can cause the following

Abusive nature
Aggression
Anger
Bad manners
Compassion and love
Compulsive behaviors
Does not like to make friends
Does not trust anyone
Easily upset
Excessive laughing or crying

Guilt
Hostility
Insecurity
Joy
Lack of emotions
overexcitement
Lack of love and compassion
Sadness
Self-confidence
Type A personality

Essential Nutrients to Strengthen the Heart Meridian

Calcium, vitamin C, vitamin E, fatty acids, selenium, potassium, sodium, iron, and B complex.

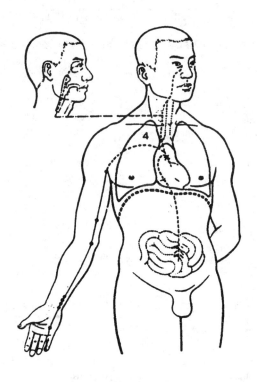

FIGURE 7-5

THE HEART MERIDIAN (HT)

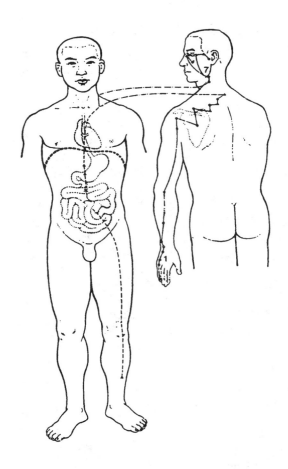

FIGURE 7-6

THE SMALL INTESTINE MERIDIAN (SI)

THE SMALL INTESTINE MERIDIAN (SI)

Energy disturbance in the small intestine meridian affecting physical and physiological levels can give rise to the following symptoms

Abdominal fullness
Abdominal pain
Acne on the upper back
Bad breath
Bitter taste in the mouth
Constipation
Diarrhea
Distention of lower abdomen
Dry stool
Frozen shoulder
Knee pain
Night sweats

Numbness of the back of the
    shoulder and arm
Numbness of the mouth and
    tongue
Pain along the lateral aspect
    of the shoulder and arm
Pain in the neck
Pain radiating around the waist
Shoulder pain
Sore throat
Stiff neck

Energy disturbance in the small intestine meridian affecting the cellular level can cause the following

Insecurity
Absentmindedness
Becoming too involved with
    details
Day dreaming
Easily annoyed
Emotional instability
Feeling of abandonment
Feeling shy
Having a tendency to be
    introverted and easily hurt
Irritability

Excessive joy or lack of
    joy
Lacking- confidence
Over excitement
Paranoia
Poor concentration
Sadness
Sighing
Sorrow
Suppressing deep
    sorrow

Essential Nutrients to Strengthen the Small Intestine Meridian

Vitamin B complex, vitamin D, vitamin E, acidophilus, yoghurt, fibers, fatty acids, wheat germ and whole grains.

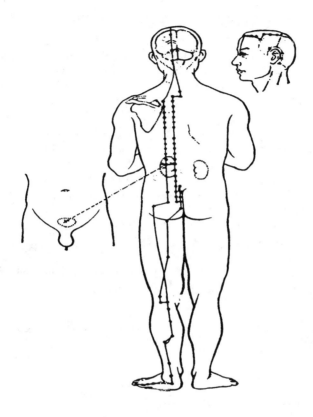

FIGURE 7-7
URINARY BLADDER MERIDIAN (UB)

URINARY BLADDER MERIDIAN (UB)

<u>Energy disturbance in the Urinary Bladder meridian affecting physical and physiological levels can give rise to the following symptoms</u>

Arthritis of little finger & toe
Bloody urine
Burning or painful urination
Chills and fever
Disease of the eye
Frequent urination
Headaches at the back of the neck
Loss of bladder control
Lower backache and stiffness
lower abdominal discomfort
Mental disorders
Muscle wasting
Nasal congestion

Pain in the inner canthus
Pain and/or spasms along back
  of the leg, foot and lateral
    part of the sole & toes
Pain in the ankle (lateral part)
Pain along the meridian
Retention of urine
Sciatic neuralgia
Spasm behind the knee
Spasms of the calf muscles
Stiff neck
Weakness in the rectum and
  rectal muscle

<u>Energy disturbance in the bladder meridian affecting the cellular level can cause the following</u>

Fright
Sadness
Disturbing and impure
  thoughts
Annoyed
Fearful
Unhappy

Frustrated
Highly irritable
Impatient
Inefficient
Insecure
Reluctant
Restless

<u>Essential Nutrients to Strengthen the Bladder Meridian</u>

Vitamin C, A, E, B complex, especially B_1, calcium, amino acids and trace minerals.

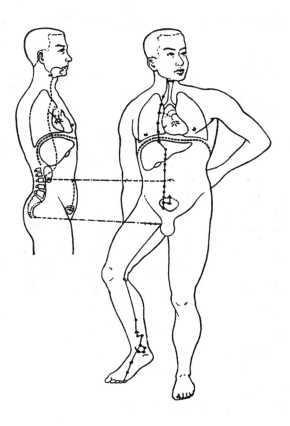

FIGURE 7-8

THE KIDNEY MERIDIAN (KI)

THE KIDNEY MERIDIAN (KI)

Energy disturbance in the kidney meridian affecting physical and physiological levels can give rise to the following symptoms

Bags under the eyes
Blurred vision
Burning or painful urination
Chronic diarrhea
Coldness in the back
Cold feet
Crave salt
Dark circles under the eyes
Dryness of the mouth
Excessive sleeping
Excessive salivation
Excessive thirst
Facial edema
Fatigue
Fever with chills
Frequent urination
Impotence
Irritability
Light- headedness
Lower backache

Motor impairment
Muscular atrophy of the foot
Nagging mild asthma
Nausea
Pain in the sole of the foot
Pain in the posterior aspect of the leg or thigh
Pain in the ears
Poor memory
Poor concentration
Poor appetite
Puffy eyes
Ringing in the ears
Sore throat
Spasms of the ankle and feet
Swelling in the legs
Swollen ankles and vertigo

Energy disturbance in the kidney meridian affecting the cellular level can cause the following

Fear
Terror
Caution
Confused

Indecision
Paranoia
Seeks attention
Unable to express feelings

Essential Nutrients to Strengthen the Kidney Meridian

Vitamins A, E, B, essential fatty acids, amino acids, sodium chloride (table salt), trace minerals, calcium and iron.

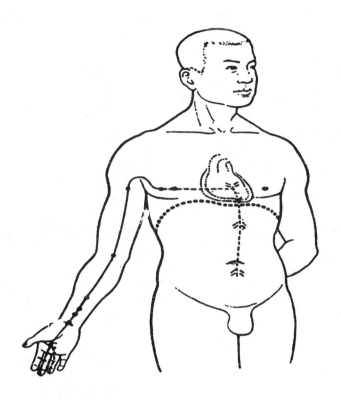

FIGURE 7-9

THE PERICARDIUM MERIDIAN (PC)

THE PERICARDIUM MERIDIAN (PC)

Energy disturbance in the pericardium meridian affecting physical and physio-logical levels can give rise to the following symptoms

Chest pain
Contracture of the arm or elbow
Excessive appetite
Fainting spells
Flushed face
Frozen shoulder
Fullness in the chest
Heaviness in the chest
Hot palms and soles
Impaired speech
Irritability
Motor impairment of the tongue
Nausea
Nervousness
Pain in the anterior part of
  the thigh
Pain in the eyes
Pain in the medial part of the
  knee
Palpitation
Restricting movements
Sensation of hot or cold
Slurred speech
Spasms of the elbow and
  arm

Energy Disturbance in the Pericardium Meridian Affecting the Cellular Level Can Cause the Following

Extreme joy
Fear of heights
Heaviness in the chest due
  to emotional overload
Heaviness in the head
Hurt
Imbalance in sexual energy
  like never having enough
  sex
In some cases no desire for sex
Jealousy
Light sleep with dreams
Manic disorders
Over- excitement
Regret
Sexual tension
Shock
Stubbornness
Various phobias

Essential Nutrients to Strengthen the Pericardium Meridian

Vitamin E, Vitamin C, Chromium, Manganese, Lotus seed, and Trace Minerals.

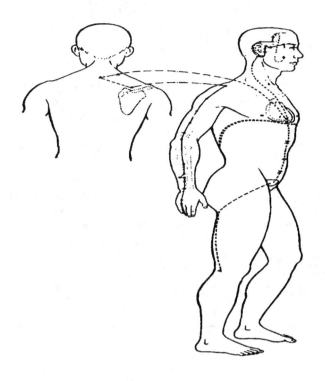

FIGURE 7-10

THE TRIPLE WARMER MERIDIAN (TW)

THE TRIPLE WARMER MERIDIAN (TW)

Energy disturbance in the triple warmer meridian affecting physical and physiological levels can give rise to the following symptoms

Abdominal pain
Always feels hungry even
   after eating a full meal
Constipation
Deafness
Distention
Dysuria
Edema
Enuresis
Excessive thirst
Excessive hunger
Fever in the late evening
Frequent urination
Indigestion

Hardness and fullness in
   the lower abdomen
Pain in the medial part of
   the knee
Pain in the shoulder and
   upper arm
Pain behind the ear
Pain in the cheek and jaw
Redness in the eye
Shoulder pain
Swelling and pain in the
   throat
Vertigo

Energy disturbance in the triple warmer meridian affecting the cellular level
can cause the following

Depression
Deprivation
Despair
Emptiness

Excessive Emotion
Grief
Hopelessness
Phobias

Essential nutrients to strengthen the triple warmer meridian

Iodine, trace minerals, vitamin C, calcium, fluoride, radish, onion, zinc,
vanadium, and water.

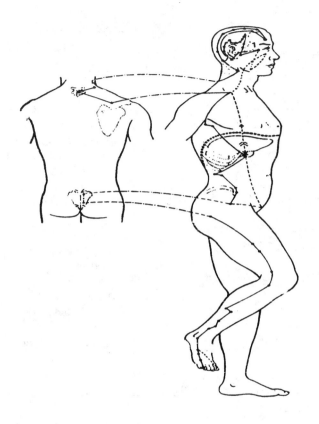

FIGURE 7-11

THE GALL BLADDER MERIDIAN (GB)

THE GALL BLADDER MERIDIAN (GB)

Energy disturbance in the gall bladder meridian affecting physical and physiological levels can give rise to the following symptoms

A heavy sensation in the right upper part of the abdomen
Abdominal bloating
Alternating fever and chills
Ashen complexion
Bitter taste in the mouth
Burping after meals
Chills
Deafness
Dizziness
Fever
Headaches on the sides of the head
Heartburn after fatty foods
Hyperacidity
Moving arthritis
Pain in the jaw
Nausea with fried foods
Pain in the eye
Pain in the hip
Pain and cramps along the anterolateral wall
Poor digestion of fats
Sciatic neuralgia
Sighing
Stroke-like condition
Swelling in the submaxillary region
Tremors
Twitching
Vision disturbances
Vomiting
Yellowish complexion

Energy Disturbance in the Gall Bladder Meridian Affecting the Cellular Level Can Cause the Following

Aggression
Complaining all the time
Rage
Fearful, finding faults with others
Unhappiness.

Essential Nutrients to Strengthen the Gall Bladder Meridian

Vitamin A, apples, lemon, calcium, linoleic acids and oleic acids (for example, pine nuts, olive oil).

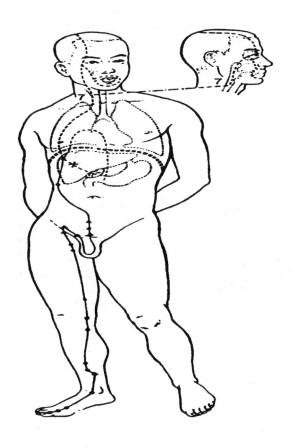

FIGURE 7-12

THE LIVER MERIDIAN (LIV)

THE LIVER MERIDIAN (LIV)

Energy disturbance in the liver meridian affecting physical and physiological levels can give rise to the following symptoms

Abdominal pain
Blurred vision
Dark urine
Dizziness
Enuresis
Bright colored bleeding during
  menses
Feeling of obstruction in the
  throat
Fever
Hard lumps in the upper
  abdomen
Headache at the top of the head
Hernia
Hemiplegia
Irregular menses

Jaundice
Loose stools
Pain in the intercostal region
Pain in the breasts
Pain in the lower abdomen
Paraplegia
PMS
Reproductive organ
  disturbances
Retention of urine
Seizures
Spasms in the extremities
Stroke-like condition
Tinnitus
Vertigo
Vomiting.

Energy disturbance in the liver meridian affecting the cellular level can cause the following

Anger
Irritability
Aggression
Assertion

Rage
Shouting
Talking loud
Type A personality

Essential Nutrients to Strengthen the Liver Meridian

Beets, green vegetables, vitamin A, trace minerals, vitamin F

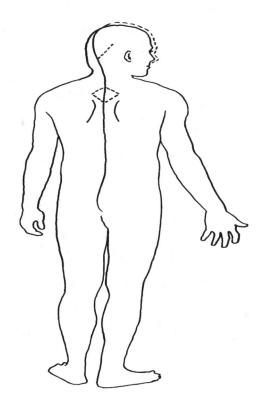

FIGURE 7-13

THE GOVERNING VESSEL MERIDIAN (GV)

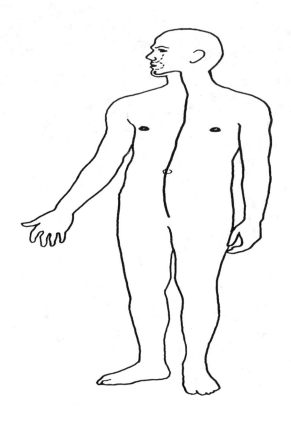

FIGURE 7-14

THE CONCEPTION VESSEL MERIDIAN (CV, REN)

THE GOVERNING VESSEL MERIDIAN (GV)

Energy disturbance in the governing vessel meridian affecting physical, physiological and psychological levels can give rise to various mixed symptoms of other yang meridians.

This channel supplies the brain and spinal region and intersects the liver channel at the vertex. Obstruction of its Chi may result in symptoms such as stiffness and pain along the spinal column. Deficient Chi in the channel may produce a heavy sensation in the head, vertigo and shaking. Energy blockages in this meridian (which passes through the brain) may be responsible for certain mental disorders. Febrile diseases are commonly associated with the governing vessel channel and because one branch of the channel ascends through the abdomen, when the channel is unbalanced, its Chi rushes upward toward the heart. Symptoms such as colic, constipation, enuresis, hemorrhoids and functional infertility may result.

THE CONCEPTION VESSEL MERIDIAN (CV, REN)

Energy disturbance in the conception vessel meridian affecting physical, physiological and psychological levels can give rise to various mixed symptoms of other yin meridians.

The conception vessel channel is the confluence of the Yin channels. Therefore, abnormality along the conception vessel channel will appear principally in pathological symptoms of the Yin channels, especially symptoms associated with the liver and kidneys. Its function is closely related with pregnancy and, therefore, has intimate links with the kidneys and uterus. If its Chi is deficient, infertility or other disorders of the urogenital system may result. Leukorrhea, irregular menstruation, colic, low libido, impotency, male and female infertility are associated with the conception vessel channel.

Any allergen can cause blockage in one or more meridians at the same time. If it is causing blockages in only one meridian, the patient may demonstrate symptoms related to that particular meridian. The intensity of the symptoms will depend on the severity of the blockage. The patient may suffer from one symptom, many symptoms or all the symptoms of this blocked meridian.

Sometimes a patient can have many meridians blocked at the same time. In such cases, the patient may demonstrate a variety of symptoms, one symptom from each meridian or many symptoms from certain meridians and one or two from other. Some patients with blockage in one meridian can demonstrate just one symptom from the list, but it may be with great intensity.

Some people, even though they have energy disturbances in multiple meridians, may not show any symptoms. Such patients might have a better immune system than others. Variations with all these possibilities can make diagnosis difficult in some cases.

8

HELPING YOUR CHILD

Most of the cases of autism spectrum disorders I have seen suffer from various sensitivities and allergies and fall into the category of allergy-related autism. Children with different stages of autistic behaviors respond differently. I have treated autistic patients ranging in age from 3 to 31 years old. The younger we begin the treatments, the faster the results.

There is no known pharmacotherapy available for autism. Symptomatic treatments are given by other medical practitioners to autistic children. If they are hyperactive, drugs are given to calm them. If they are too passive stimulants are given. These drugs may help the children to adjust to situations. However, they may not have long term effects. In fact if the child is allergic to the drug, it can do more damage to the already affected brain.

During the past decade many controversies and concerns have been raised about the use of medication for autistic children because most children with autism have such severe allergies that they exhibit varying symptoms in varying degrees. As a result they respond differently to medications. Most autistic children are unable to report allergic reactions to their parents or caretakers due to their inability to communicate. If the parents and/or caretakers are taught NST (MRT), parents can screen the medication for possible allergies before they administer it to the children. There is no harm in using drugs to handle appropriate situations as long as the person who administers the drug knows its purpose and the condition of the patient.

We now know that most of the causes of autism are in fact, undiagnosed allergies, which when left untreated can become serious health problems in the future. An allergy is an over-reaction of the immune system. In NAET, allergies are viewed from a holistic perspective based on Oriental medical principles.

When the body, or the electromagnetic field of the body, makes contact with an allergen, it causes blockages in the energy pathways called meridians. Put in another way, we can say, it disrupts the normal flow of energy through the body's electrical circuits. The energy flows in the body through the nerve pathways with the help of various neurotransmitters. This energy blockage causes interference in appropriate neurotransmitter production and proper utilization causing poor communication between the brain, different parts of the body and the nervous system. The obstructed energy flow is the first step in a chain of events, which can develop into an allergic response. An allergic reaction is the result of continuous energy imbalances in the body, leading to a diminished state of health in one or more organs.

The spleen, kidney, and liver meridians are most commonly affected in autistic people. The other meridians and related organs receiving disturbed energy flow are lungs, stomach, heart, gall bladder, small intestine, and large intestine. NAET uses NST to test the allergens and to detect blockages in meridians - Refer to Chapter Three. In some cases, all of the above meridians are affected by allergens. In others, just one or two meridians are affected with most allergens. Yet in some other cases, every allergen affects random meridian(s) without any regular pattern. NAET can treat all of these types with ease.

AN EVALUATION OF AUTISM BY NAET

♦ A thorough medical and family history, prenatal history of the mother (if she suffered from any potentially related condition or emotional trauma during pregnancy, etc.), emotional, social and environmental history (parental divorce, child abuse, death of a loved one, environmental or residential disruption, a newcomer in the family or arrival of a new sibling).

♦ Behavior ratings completed by parents and teacher.

♦ An evaluation done by the child psychologist or the treating pediatrician.

♦ A physical examination at the NAET office. This should include vital signs, NAET Autism Rating Scale, NAET Allergy Grading Instrument, NAET General Screening Device, Childhood Autism Scale, and ARI Diagnostic Checklist E2 form, etc.).

♦ Information about the commonly consumed foods and drinks, commonly used clothes, chemicals in the environment, exposure to pesticides, immunizations, vaccinations, medications, any special addictions to toys, blankets, and furniture, etc. (could be allergic to any one of them).

♦ Blood serum study for IgE specific antigens by RAST to screen sensitivities to 30 different food substances.

WESTERN TREATMENT APPROACHES

Western medical approaches for such conditions are:

In less severe cases:

♦ Behavior modification

♦ Educational modification

♦ Psychological counseling

♦ Pharmaceutical drugs

In extremely severe cases none of the above works except pharmaceutical drugs to calm them down.

Medication has proven temporarily effective to calm them down but does not provide long-term cure for many children with autism. It has been found helpful in alleviating the symptoms in some children and adults. Some autistic children suffer from seizure disorders. Such children may need medication to keep their seizures under control. If there are no side effects, it is permissible to use medication to help the child function better. But it is very important to check for an allergy to the medication before administering it. If the child is allergic to the drug, it is not going to give the expected results. In some children an allergy to drugs could make their condition worse. They may become hyper, violent, irritable beyond control, and may display unpleasant side effects like itching, hives, eczema, indigestion, bowel and bladder incontinence, bleeding from various parts of the body, etc. In such cases, medication must be stopped and should not be used again until the allergy is eliminated.

In my experience, autistic children are usually allergic to many foods and chemicals they use in their daily lives. Some children may outgrow these allergic symptoms or change their symptoms into something totally new depending on the course of the obstructed meridians on a particular day.

Even though Western medical practitioners are using thoroughly researched pharmaceutical drugs, they are chemical compounds, which can have related allergy and side effects in certain individuals. Allergic reactions and side effects have created constant fear in some people, discouraging them from using drugs. More and more people are becoming negative about taking drugs and are using natural products. Long term use of drugs can destroy the body's garbage disposal – the Liver—sometimes such damages are irreversible or very slow to reverse.

ALTERNATIVE THERAPIES

Practitioners and consumers are looking for natural means to control this disorder. Out of necessity, many alternative therapies have been developed and are available for autistic children today that produce inner calmness and serenity without the usage of drugs. Some of these commonly used therapies are given below.

BEHAVIOR MODIFICATION IN CONJUNCTION WITH:

♦ Vitamin-mineral therapy.

♦ Amino-acid therapy.

♦ Fatty Acid therapy.

♦ Various detoxification programs to remove toxins and parasites.

♦ Herbal supplementation, biofeedback, and living in a chemical-free environment.

♦ Diet management (removing sugar, artificial sweeteners, corn, gluten, milk, dairy products, yeast, food additives, food colors, and carbonated water from the diet entirely).

♦ Providing regular chiropractic and acupuncture or acupressure treatments.

♦ Regular therapeutic massages and saunas.

♦ Encouraging Yoga and meditation practices.

♦ Magnetic therapy.

♦ Engaging in regular sports and exercise programs.

♦ NAET treatments.

Through various studies, clinical trials and case reports, NAET has proven to be the most effective alternative therapy to reduce or eliminate autism by eliminating the causes of autism permanently. In most cases, the causes were their undiagnosed allergies to food and environmental factors.

NAET can bring a balance between liver and spleen meridians. through NAET treatments we are able to control and eliminate allergies and allergic reactions to all known allergens from the child's surroundings, often giving permanent relief from the symptoms of allergies permitting the child to eat, drink, and use the items the child was allergic to once, without giving rise to future allergic reactions. When the child becomes nonreactive to what were previously allergens then the child will begin to absorb the nutrients from the daily food he/she consumes. These nutrients will help repair the brain and nervous system and help to restore or restart the brain functions. When NAET treatments are completed for all known allergies, the autistic child will be free of his/her autism and be able to lead a normal life again.

THE STEPS OF NAET TREATMENT

Step-1: Isolate the offending allergen with the help of NST and NAET Allergy Grading Instrument. Evaluation is also done via standardized laboratory tests for IgE specific antigens via RAST (enzyme-linked immunozorbant assay), and all other checklists mentioned in chapter 3.

Step-2: When the allergen is isolated using any of the above measures, mild acupressure is administered by the NAET practitioner using specific NAET acupressure technique on pre-determined acupuncture points on the specific acupuncture meridians.

Step-3: Complete avoidance of the treated allergen for 25 hours following the treatment (or otherwise determined by the practitioner) is necessary to imprint the new memory about the harmlessness of the allergen in the child's brain. After 25 hours, the practitioner needs to retest the treated allergen to determine the completeness of the treatment. In most cases, it takes one treatment per single group or a single allergen (one office visit) to reduce or eliminate the allergy towards one single allergen, if the treatment is administered properly and the 25-hour avoidance period is properly followed. In some cases, especially in severe cases of autism it may take a few office visits (three or four) per item to desensitize completely. The child will be able to use the treated allergen without any adverse reactions when the allergen has been completely desensitized using NAET.

The most effective treatment option for allergies in traditional medicine until now has been complete avoidance of the offending allergens. What can one avoid if one is allergic to everything around him/her? I have found most autistic children reacting to everything in their lives; everything they eat, drink, touch, breathe, play with, and even allergy to their parents, siblings, caretakers, sitters, etc. NAET can desensitize the child(ren) for all of the above. But it takes many office visits since desensitization can be done for only one item per visit. Usually most children with fair amount of allergies will take 100 office visits or more to get normalized.

If the children are severely autistic they can take more than 100 to 150 office visits before they become functional. Even if it takes several office visits, there is a hope at the end of the tunnel with NAET.

Can you imagine keeping your child on a diet, month after month and year after year, especially if that diet contains no egg, soy, fruits, vegetables, wheat, corn, rice, sugar, chocolate, fats, hamburgers, French fries, ice cream, milk, butter, oils, gluten, MSG, spices, whiten-all, food additives, carbonated drinks, and food colorings, etc.? Impossible! That's where NAET comes in. NAET will accommodate our "21st century life-styles." It doesn't mean that you should go out of your way to feed your child with any junk food available after completing NAET treatments. You and your child should eat normal, healthy, nutritious food as much as possible. Unhealthy but commonly eaten zesty foods like pastry, cream pies, carbonated drinks, etc. should be consumed once in a while only.

NAET can remove the adverse effect of any allergic food in the body and create homeostasis in the presence of the offending allergen (without avoiding it for life). During the NAET treatment, your brain will create a new friendly memory toward the allergen and will imprint and store this new memory in your memory bank. During this process, the old memory of the allergen's adverse effect is erased or forgotten. After completion of the NAET treatment, the allergen becomes a non-allergen, and an irritant becomes a non-irritant to your energy field. The body will learn to relax naturally in the presence of the new friendly substance. When the brain is not frightened about the contact with the new harmless substance (previously an allergen), natural calmness comforts the brain.

In the presence of such items, the brain will not panic any more. It does not have to alert the immune system for fight or flight causing allergic reactions, anaphylactic shocks or other chronic pains and illnesses as a result of brain and nervous system facing continuous fight or flight situation on a daily basis.

So far I have not found any record or heard of any report on any other medical treatment that can eliminate allergies and allergic reactions permanently to the treated allergen(s) and be able to free the body from myraid illnesses that started with allergies or allergic reactions.

SUPPORTIVE TREATMENTS

NOURISH THE BRAIN

Start the day with this special rejuvenating brain tonic.

Make sure the autistic person is allergy-free to the following ingredients before you prepare the food. If you find an allergy to one or more items, please exclude them from the drink until you clear the allergy to them. Each of these nutrients nourishes the respective meridians and associated organs and helps to enhance the functions of the area by eliminating the energy blockages in those meridians.

1/4 teaspoon barley green powder (St, Sp, brain)

6 ounces of apple juice (Liver, GB, Colon)

1/4 teaspoon of freshly ground flax seed powder (GB, blood vessels)

1 pinch of cinnamon (Lu, PC & TW)

1 tablespoonful of honey (brain & nervous system)

50 mgs B6 (brain & nervous system)

50 mgs B complex (brain & nervous system)

2 drops grape seed oil (brain)

2 drops olive leaf extract or 1 capsule (immune system)

1 drop oregano oil (blood purifier)

1 pinch of Epsom salt (liver, colon, brain & nervous system)

1 ounce cranberry juice (kid & UB)

1 scoop Endfatigue Enfusion (multivitamin - mineral formula from www.vitality 101.com) or you may substitute any well balanced multivitamin-mineral formula).

2 tablespoonsful of prune juice (SI & LI).

Blend all the ingredients and drink three ounces twice a day preferably in the morning after breakfast and before going to bed.

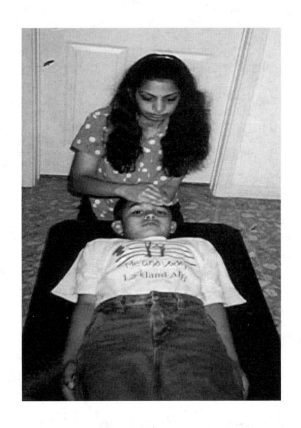

FIGURE 8-1
BRAIN RELEASE

BRAIN RELEASE

The child lies on his/her back. The mother/helper sits next to his/her head, supporting the head in her left palm as in diagram 8-1. Find the point just above the eyebrows on the forehead and with the right palm gently swipe towards the top of the head while the child breathes in. When you get to the top of the head, gently release the hand and the child breathes out. Do this swiping massage technique three times. Turn the head to one side. Support the head on the bottom side with one palm, cupping the ear with the supporting palm (eg. the left ear and side of the head), massage gently up the side of the cheek in front of the opposite ear (the side facing up, here for example. in front of the right ear), while the child breathes in. Do both sides this way three times each. Then cradle the head in both hands and hold it there for 30 seconds then release it.

Finally, massage or rub the vertex or the top of the head for 30 seconds as in Fig. 8-2. This massage helps to get rid of the toxins from the brain.

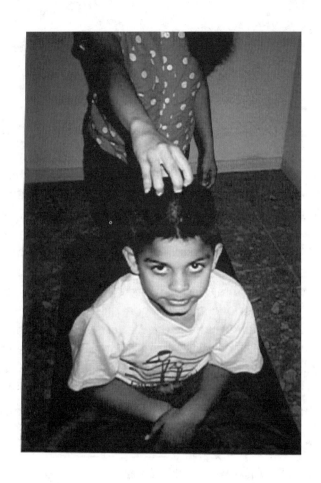

FIGURE 8-2
VERTEX MASSAGE

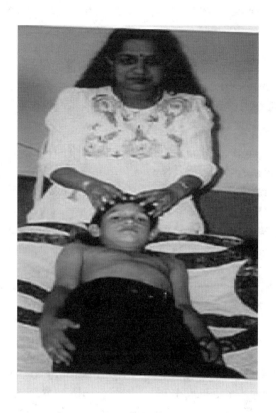

FIGURE 8-3

THE CEPHALIC RUB

According to Chinese medical principles, all Yang meridians pass through the head traveling close to the superficial level reporting each and every energetic activity of every instant to the brain. All Yin meridians also pass through the head at a deeper level supporting and confirming the finding of their counterparts, Yang meridians, according to *Tang Dynasty physician Sun Si-Mo,"The three hundred connecting channels all rise to the head."* When you massage the whole head gently with a kneading movement, you are in fact invigorating all the energy meridians forcing the energy blockages to come out of the meridians and helping the energy to circulate freely through the energy pathways.

A-fifteen-minute massage, once every other day will help to nourish and stabilize the brain. After the head massage the person should lie down flat for an hour allowing the energy to concentrate in the brain tissues. The best time to do this head massage is before bedtime. The massage can be done using massage olive oil and/or coconut oil. Pioneer medical experts believed massaging with nourishing nutrients would help to nourish the brain faster. Massaging once a week with clarified butter, cooked mung bean paste or cooked brown rice with a few drops of grape seed oil and olive oil is beneficial in some cases.

Method: Cook brown rice or mung bean with the skin still on. After bringing it to room temperature blend it with a few drops of grape seed oil and olive oil. Massage the whole head for 15 minutes with this nutrient paste once a week. Wait for 30 minutes to an hour, then wash the head thoroughly and dry it.

THYMUS STIMULATION

Thymus gland stimulation helps to improve the immune system reducing the allergic reactions. Since autistic children

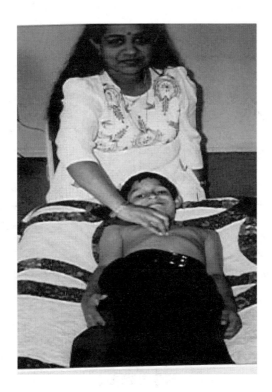

FIGURE 8-4

THYMUS STIMULATION

have poor immune systems and severe allergies, thymus stimulation has been very helpful in improving their immune system. A simple clockwise, gentle massage on the thymus gland as given in figure 8-4 for 1 minute daily preferably in the morning will be helpful.

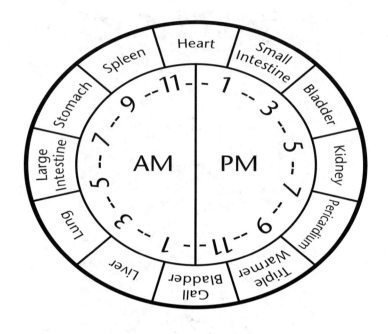

FIGURE 8-5

MERIDIAN CLOCK

When the energy is blocked in a certain meridian, the effect of the blockage can be felt at its worst during the corresponding time of the meridian. When a person does not feel good, look at the meridian clock to find the corresponding meridian according to the time. Find the meridian pathway from Chapter 7 and apply gentle strokes using your finger pads along the flow of meridian from the beginning point towards the end point of the meridian to guide the blocked energy into the circulation. When the blockage is manually pushed forward, energy circulation will be re-established and the person will feel better.

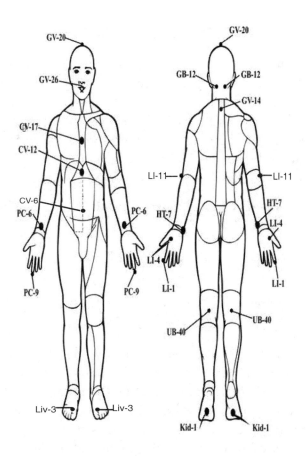

FIGURE 8-6

RESUSCITATION POINTS

ACUPRESSURE RESUSCITATION

Some commonly used acupuncture points, and their uses to help in emergency situations, are given below. Massage these points shown in the previous figure gently with the finger pads for one minute each. Please refer to the appropriate meridians in Chapter 10 of my book, *Say Good-bye to Illness* or refer to the textbooks on acupuncture in the bibliography if you would like to learn more about these points.

POINTS TO HELP WITH MEDICAL EMERGENCIES

1. Fainting: GV-20, GV-26, GB-12, LI-1, PC-9, Kid-1
2. Nausea: CV-12, PC-6, Ht-7
3. Backache: GV-26, UB-40
4. Fatigue: CV-6, LI-1, CV-17, Liv-3
5. Fever: LI-11, GV-14

Stimulate these points on figure 8-6 by massaging them clockwise one at a time (from right to left on the patient's body) as you need them to control acute symptoms. Patients will usually respond within 30 seconds to one minute of stimulating these points. If someone is slow to respond, it is OK to massage for three to five minutes. But please stop and evaluate the condition of the patient every 30 seconds.

Do not hesitate to call for emergency help (911), if you ever need it. For more information on revival techniques, refer to Chapter 3, pages 570 to 573, in *"Acupuncture: A Comprehensive Text,"* by Shanghai College of Traditional Medicine, Eastland Press, or refer to my book, *"Living Pain Free with Acupressure."* It is available at various bookstores and at our **website (naet.com).**

9

NAET ALLERGENS

C hildren and adults suffering from the symptoms
of autism are usually allergic to the following food
groups, which are listed according to their importance
to the body. It is necessary to follow the restricted diet and your
NAET specialist's instructions carefully during the 25 hours after
the treatment in order to pass for the allergen being treated. You
may also refer to the "NAET Guide Book" for more information
on NAET treatments and specific instructions to follow during
the 25 hour-avoidance period.

Most autistic children and adults can get their symptoms under
control when they complete the NAET basic 30-45 groups of
allergens successfully. Some autistic children and adults with mild
to moderate symptoms may show marked improvements after they
complete just five basic groups of allergens. But it is to their
advantage to complete the 35- 40 groups of allergens before they
stop the treatments.

After treating each group of allergens, after 25 hours, such item should be tested individually to be certain that the treatment has been completed. Some children may need repeated treatments on egg white, egg yolk, etc.

The 25 hour-food restriction should be observed on all treatments. Autistic children tend to fall out of treatments when the allergens are not avoided for 25 hours. In some children I have observed that it is necessary to avoid the treated food allergen for 30 hours. This may be due to the fact that autistic children have extremely fatigued and diminished brain function.

1. Egg Mix (egg white, egg yolk, chicken, and tetracycline, feather.)

You may have brown or white rice, pasta without eggs, vegetables, fruits, milk products, oils, beef, pork, fish, coffee, juice, soft drinks, water, and tea.

To be checked individually: egg white, egg yolk, chicken, feather, tetracycline.

2. Calcium mix (breast milk, cow's milk, goat's milk, milk albumin, casein, coumarin, lactic acid and calcium)

You may have cooked rice, cooked fruits and vegetables (like potato, squash, green beans, yams, cauliflower, sweet potato), chicken, red meat, and drink coffee, tea without milk, and distilled or boiled, cooled water.

To be checked individually: Milk albumin, milk casein.

3. Vitamin C (fruits, vegetables, vinegar, citrus, and berry. Check them individually.)

You may have cooked white or brown rice, pasta without sauce, boiled or poached eggs, baked or broiled chicken, fish, red meat, brown toast, deep fried food, French fries, salt, oils, coffee without milk, and water. When the vitamin C treatment is over it is advised to bring fresh green leafy vegetable and other vegetables to get checked individually and treat for them if necessary. After completing the treatments for vegetables and leafy green vegetables, plenty of them should be included in the child's daily diet.

4. B complex vitamins (17 B vitamins. Check them individually.)
You may have cooked white rice, cauliflower raw or cooked, well cooked or deep fried fish, salt, white sugar, black coffee, French fries, and purified, non allergic water. Rice should be washed well before cooking. It should be cooked in lots of water and drained well to remove the fortified vitamins. After successfully completing the treatment for vitamin B complex (should be checked for individual B vitamins, if necessarey should be treated individually), children should be supplemented with vitamin B complex and diet should include whole grains.

5. Sugar Mix (cane sugar, corn sugar, maple sugar, grape sugar, rice sugar, brown sugar, beet sugar, fructose, molasses, honey, dextrose, glucose, and maltose.)
You may have white rice, pasta, vegetables, vegetable oils, meats, eggs, chicken, water, coffee, tea without milk.
To be checked individually for all sugars.

6. Iron Mix (animal and vegetable sources, beef, pork, lamb, raisin, date, and broccoli.)
You may have white rice without iron fortification, sour dough bread without iron, cauliflower, white potato, chicken, light green vegetables (white cabbage, iceberg lettuce, white squash), yellow squash, distilled water and orange juice.

7. Vitamin A (animal and vegetable source, beta carotene, fish and shellfish.)
You may have cooked rice, pasta, potato, cauliflower, red apples, chicken, water, and coffee without milk.

To be checked individually: fish mix, shellfish mix, beta carotene.

8. Mineral Mix (magnesium, manganese, phosphorus, selenium, zinc, copper, cobalt, chromium, molybdenum, trace minerals, gold, mercury, lead, cadmium, aluminum, arsenic, copper, gold, silver, vanadium and fluoride.)

You may use only distilled water for washing, drinking, and showering. You may eat only cooked rice, vegetables, fruits, meats, eggs, milk, coffee, and tea. No root vegetables.

9. Magnesium

Avoid green vegetables and whole grains.

10. Salt Mix (sodium and sodium chloride.)

You may use distilled water for drinking and washing, cooked rice, fresh vegetables and fruits (except celery, carrots, beets, artichokes, romaine lettuce, and watermelon) meats, chicken, and sugars.

11. Corn Mix (blue corn, yellow corn, cornstarch, cornsilk, corn syrup.)

You may eat only steamed vegetables, steamed rice, broccoli, baked chicken, and meats. You may drink water, tea and/or coffee without cream or sugar.

12. Grain Mix (wheat, gluten, gliadin, coumarin, rye, oats, millet, barley, and rice.)

You may eat vegetables, fruits, meats, milk, and drink water. Avoid all products with gluten.

To be checked for: wheat, gluten, gliadin, coumarin, corn, oats, millet, barley, rye, and rice.

13. Artificial Sweeteners (Sweet and Low, Equal, Saccharine, Twin, and Aspartame.)

You may eat anything without artificial sweeteners. Use freshly prepared items only.

14. Yeast Mix (brewer's yeast, and bakers yeast, tortula yeast, acidophilus, yogurt, and whey.)

To be individually checked: brewer's yeast, baker's yeast, whey, yogurt, and acidophilus.

You may have vegetables, egg, meat, chicken, and fish. No fruits, no sugar products. Drink distilled water.

15. Stomach acid (Hydrochloric acid.)

You may eat raw and steamed vegetables, cooked dried beans, eggs, oils, clarified butter, and milk.

16. Base (digestive juice from the intestinal tract contains various digestive enzymes: amylase, protease, lipase, maltase, peptidase, bromelain, cellulase, sucrase, papain, lactase, gluco-amylase, and alpha galactosidase.)

You may eat sugars, starches, breads, and meats.

17. Neurotransmitters: acetylcholine, nor-epinephrine, dopamine, and serotonin.

18. Immunizations and Vaccinations: either you received or your parent received before you were born. Test them individually and if found treat them individually.

MMR: (measles, mumps, rubella), DPT: (diphtheria, pertussis, tetanus), Polio vaccine, Small pox, Chicken pox, Influenza, hepatitis-B, hepatitis C.)

Each one of them should be checked and treated individually if tested to be an allergen. Nothing to avoid while treating for these except infected persons or recently inoculated persons if there are any near you. MMR and DPT should be treated for the individual components since allergic reactions to these vaccines are causing imbalances in the brain in many children.

19. Pesticides (malathion, termite control chemicals, or regular pesticides.)

Avoid meats, uncooked vegetables and fruits, grasses, trees and flowers, public areas where pesticides, ant sprays, insecticides, and other pesticides have been sprayed.

20. Alcohol (candy, ice cream, liquid medication in alcohol, and alcohol.)

Whether or not you drink alcohol, your body needs and makes it. Alcohol is made from refined starches and other forms of sugars. Many people are allergic to sugar and thus alcohol.
You may eat vegetables, meats, fish, eggs, and chicken. Avoid hair-spray, after shave, homeopathic remedies with alcohol.

Collect different food groups from every meal and treat for the mixture of breakfast, lunch and dinner. Collect this combined food sample at least four times a month and treat using NAET.

21. Chocolate Mix (coffee, chocolate, caffeine, tannic acid, cocoa, cocoa butter, and carob.)

You may consume anything that has no coffee, caffeine, chocolate and/or carob.

22. Nut Mix 1 (peanuts, black walnuts, or English walnuts.)
You may eat any foods that do not contain the nuts listed above including their oils and butter.

Nut Mix 2 (cashew, almonds, pecan, Brazil nut, hazelnut, mac adamia nut, and sunflower seeds.)

You may eat foods that do not contain the nuts listed above including their oils and butters.

23. Bacteria Mix (eat cooked foods and drink boiled cooled water)

24. Virus Mix/Parasites (avoidance - same as bacteria mix)

25. Spice Mix 1 (ginger, cardamom, cinnamon, cloves, nutmeg, garlic, cumin, fennel, coriander, turmeric, saffron, and mint.)

You may use all foods and products without these items.

Spice Mix 2 (peppers, red pepper, black pepper, green pepper, jalapeno, banana peppers, anise seed, basil, bay leaf, caraway seed, chervil, cream of tartar, dill, fenugreek, horseradish, mace, MSG, mustard, onion, oregano.)

You may eat or use all foods and food products without the above listed spices.

26. Fat mix: Animal Fats (butter, lard, chicken fat, beef fat, lamb fat, and fish oil.)

You may use anything other than the above including vegetable oils.

Vegetable Fats and vitamin F(corn oil, canola oil, peanut oil, linseed oil, sunflower oil, palm oil, flax seed oil, grape seed oil, evening primrose oil, borage oil, wheat germ oil and coconut oil.)

You may eat anything that does not contain vegetable oils, wheat germ oil, linseed oil, sunflower oil, soybean oil, safflower oil, peanuts and peanut oil.

27. Dried Bean Mix (dried beans, vegetable proteins, soybean, and lecithin.)

You may eat rice, pasta, vegetables, meats, eggs, and anything other than beans and bean products.

28. Amino Acids-1 (essential amino acids: lysine, methionine, leucine, threonine, valine, tryptophane, isoleucine, and phenylalanine. Each one should be checked each one and treated individually if found weak by NST)

You may eat cooked white rice, lettuce, and boiled chicken.

Amino Acids 2 (non essential amino acids: alanine, arginine, aspartic acid, carnitine citrulline, cysteine, glutamic acid, glycine, histidine, ornithine, proline, serine, taurine, and tyrosine. Should be checked each one and treated individually if found weak by NST)

You may eat cooked white rice, boiled beef (corned beef), and iceberg lettuce.

Dimethyl Glycine

You may eat white rice, white flour pasta, lettuce, oils and clarified butter.

29. RNA, DNA, nuclear proteins and combinations.
   Nothing to avoid.

30. Hormones (estrogen, progesterone, testosterone)
   You may eat vegetables, fruits, grains, chicken, and fish.

31. Food additives (sulfates, nitrates, BHT, whiten-all.)
You cannot eat hot dogs or any pre-packaged food. Eat anything made at home from scratch.

32. Food colorings (different food colors in many sources like: ice cream, candy, cookie, gums, drinks, spices, other foods, and/ or lipsticks, etc.)
You may eat foods that are freshly prepared. Avoid carrots, natural spices, beets, berries, frozen green leafy vegetables like spinach.

33. Night-shade vegetables (bell pepper, onion, eggplant, potato, okra, tomato (fruits, sauces, and drinks.)

Avoid eating these vegetables.

34. Starch Complex (Grains, root vegetables.)

You may have all vegetables except root vegetables, grains, yogurt, meats, chicken, and fish.

Refined starches are used as a thickening agent in sauces and drinks. Many people are allergic to starches. Refined starches should be avoided.

35. Heavy metals (Lead, mercury, arsenic, antimony, zinc, cadmium, copper, siver, gold, aluminum, sulfur)

36. Mercury   (Avoid eating fish and all mercury products)

37. Thymeresol, amalgam

38. Drugs: Any drugs given in infancy, during childhood or taken by the mother during pregnancy.

Antibiotics (check Individual antibiotics), sedatives, laxatives and recreational drugs.

39. Baking powder/ Baking soda (in baked goods, toothpaste, and/or detergents, yogurt, cosmetics.)

Avoid any items with baking powder and baking soda. You may eat or use anything that does not contain baking powder or baking soda including fresh fruits, vegetables, fats, meat, and chicken.

40. Carbohydrates (Avoid all type of carbohydrates)

41. School work materials (crayons, coloring paper and books, inks, pencils, crayons, glue, play dough, other arts and craft materials.)

Avoid using them or contacting them. Wear a pair of gloves if you have to go near them.

42. Fabrics (daily wear, sleep attire, towels, bed linens, blankets, formaldehyde. Check cotton, polyester, acrylic, rayon, etc. individually.)

Treat each kind of fabric separately and avoid the particular cloth or kind of cloth for 25 hours.

43. Water (drinking water, tap water, filtered water, city water, lake water, rain water, ocean water, and river water.)

People can react to any water. Treat them as needed and avoid the item treated. Drink boiled cooled water during 25 hours following the treatment.

44. Chemicals (chlorine, swimming pool water, detergents, fabric softeners, soaps, cleaning products, shampoos, lipsticks, and cosmetics you or other family members use.) Avoid the particular chemical treated for 25 hours.

45. Plastics (toys, play or work materials, utensils, toiletries, computer key boards, and/or phone.) Avoid contact with products made from plastics during treatment. Wear a pair of cotton gloves.

46. Hypothalamus

Nothing to avoid.

47. Brain Tissue

Nothing to avoid.

48. Parts of Brain (nerve cell, glia, dendrite, axon, cranial nerves, frontal lobe, parietal lobe, temporal lobe, occipital lobe, basal ganglia, gyrus, sympathetic and parasympathetic nerves, cerebral cortex, association cortex, Rt cerebral hemisphere, Lt cerebral hemisphere, Rt thalamus, Lt thalamus, midbrain, pons, medulla, limbic system tissue, hippocampus, corpus callosum, striatum, substantia nigra, cerebellum. Check each part separately. If any part found weak by NST, that particular tissue should be treated individually. Your NAET Specialist will know how to treat for them.)

49. Other Enzymes: Secretin, melanin, cytokinine, dopamine, histamine, endorphin, enkephalin and metabolic enzymes.

50. Perfume Mix (room deodorizers, soaps, flowers, perfumes, or after-shave, etc.).
Avoid perfume and any fragrance from flowers or products containing perfume.

51. Gelatin
You may use anything that does not contain gelatin.

52. Gum Mix (Acacia, Karaya gum, Xanthine gum, black gum, sweet gum, and chewing gum).
You may eat rice, pasta, vegetables, fruits without skins, meats, eggs, and chicken; drink juice and water.

53. Paper Products (newspaper, newspaper ink, reading books, coloring books, books with colored illustrations).
Avoid the particular product that is treated.

54. Fluoride

You may use or eat fruits, poultry, meat, potato without skin, cauliflower, white rice, and yellow vegetables. You may use distilled water, drink fresh fruit juices.

55. Vitamin E
You may eat fresh fish, carrots, potato, poultry, and meat.

56. Vitamin D
You may eat fruits, vegetables, poultry, and meats.

57. Vitamin K
You may eat fish, rice, potato, poultry, and meat.

58. Insect Bites in infancy or childhood (bee stings, spider bites, or cockroach, etc.)
Treat for the individual insect and avoid it while treating.

59. Latex (shoe, sole of the shoe, elastic, rubber bands, and/or rubber bathtub toys.)
Avoid latex products.

60. Radiation (computer, television, microwave, X-ray, and the sun).
Avoid radiation of any kind.

61. Inhalants
Pollens, weeds, grasses, flowers, wood mix, room air, outside air, smog, cold (ice cube), heat (hot water in a glass bottle), dryness (heat up a piece of cotton towel on stove-top or in a microwave oven for a few seconds and put it in a glass jar with a lid to make the sample of dry heat), dampness (use a piece of wet cloth or paper towel along with a piece of ice cube in a glass jar

to make this sample), and polluted air from nearby factories (place a piece of wet cloth in a flat open plate or container in the open air for 6-8 hours where the polluted air circulates and put it in a glass jar with lid immediately after removing from the plate, to make this sample).

62. Tissues and secretions (DNA, RNA, Cell filaments, Cell proteins, nuclear proteins, thyroid hormone, pituitary hormone, pineal gland, liver, urine, blood, and saliva)

Treat these items individually if needed. Avoid touching your own body. Wear a pair of gloves for 25 hours.

63. Allergies to people: animals and pets (mother, father, care takers, cats, and dogs)

Avoid the ones you were treated for 25 hours.

64. Emotional allergies (fear, fright, frustration, anger, low self-esteem, and/or rejection, etc.)

There is nothing to avoid for emotional treatment.

65. Other substances:

Cerebrospinal fluid, blood, parasites, other foods, environmental agents, detergent, hand washing soap, bed linen, night clothes, plastic toys on the crib, remote control for television., alarm clock on the bedside table, etc. need to be checked for allergies.

After clearing the allergy to nutrients, appropriate supplementation with vitamins, minerals, herbs, enzymes etc., is necessary to make up the deficiency and promote healing. Please check with your NAET practitioner or read the guidebook for information on how to take supplements correctly.

HIDDEN TOXINS IN THE FOOD

Other common ingredients in many preparations that children may react severely to are the various gums (acacia gum, xanthine gum, karaya gum, etc.). Numerous gums are used in candy bars, yogurt, cream cheese, soft drinks, soy sauce, barbecue sauce, fast food products, macaroni and cheese, etc.

Carob, a staple in many health food products, is another item that causes brain irritability among allergic people. Many health-conscious people are turning to natural food products in which carob is used as a chocolate and cocoa substitute. It is also used as a natural coloring or stiffening agent in soft drinks, cheeses, sauces, etc. We discovered that some of the causes of "holiday flu" and suicide attempts are allergies to carob, chocolate, and turkey.

If your child has allergies you must look for these ingredients and additives in the food products you buy from the market.

Please read the labels. Manufacturers usually list these items on the cover of the product-container.

Acetic Acid (sodium acetate and sodium diacetate). This is a common food additive. This is the acid of vinegar. Acetic acid is used as an acidic flavoring agent for pickles, sauces, catsups, mayonnaise, wine, foods that are preserved in vinegar, some soft drinks, processed cheese, baked goods, cheese spreads, sweet and sour drinks and soups. It is also naturally found in apples, cocoa, coffee, wine, cheese, grapes, and other over-ripened fruits. If your child gets allergic reaction to these natural foods he/she may be allergic to acetic acid.

Agar (Seaweed extract): This is a polysaccharide that comes from several varieties of algae and it can turn like a gel if you dissolve it in water. So this is used in ice cream, jellies, preserves, icings, laxatives, used as a thickening agent in milk, cream, and used as gelatin (vegetable form). This is a safe additive, but if your child is allergic to sea foods you may need to eliminate the allergy for this.

Albumin (cow milk-albumin): Many children are allergic to albumin in the milk. Researchers have found children/people who are allergic to milk albumin are at high risk to get any of these disorders: ADD, ADHD, Autism, bipolar diseases, schizophrenia, and other allergy-related brain disorders. NAET can desensitize you for milk-albumin.

Aldicarb: It is an organic chemical water pollutant, seen often in city water. When the concentration of this chemical gets high in the city water, many people get sick with gastrointestinal disorders, like nausea, vomiting, pain, bloating, stomach flu, etc. Boiling the water for 30 minutes could help reduce the reaction. If your child is not allergic to apple cider vinegar, adding two-three drops of vinegar in eight ounces of water might help.

Alginates (Alginic acid, algin gum, ammonium, calcium, potassium, and sodium alginates, propylene glycol alginates): Most of these are natural extracts of seaweed and used in the food industry primarily as stabilizing agents.

Propylene glycol is an antifreeze. This is considered as a safe solvent, used in food preparation. Alginates help to retain water, helps to prevent ice crystal formation; helps uniform distribution of flavors in foods, add smoothness and texture to the products and are used in ice creams, custards, chocolates, chocolate milk, cheese, salad dressings, jellies, cakes, icings, jams, and soft drinks.

Aluminum Salts (alum hydroxide, alum potassium sulfate, sodium alum phosphate, alum ammonium sulfate, and alum calcium silicate).: Aluminum salts are used as a buffer in various products. This helps to balance the acidity. Used as an astringent to keep canned produce firm, to lighten food texture, and used as an anti-caking agent.

Sodium aluminum phosphate is used in baking powder and in self-rising flours. Alum is used as a clarifier for sugar and as a hardening agent. Aluminum hydroxide is used as a leavening agent in baked goods. It is a strong alkali agent that can be toxic but when used in small amounts it is fairly safe. It is also used in antiperspirants and antacids. Aluminum ammonium sulfate is used as an astringent, and neutralizing agent in baking powder and cereals. It can cause burning sensation to the mucous membranes. Overuse of aluminum products may lead to aluminum toxicity and it can affect the brain chemistry. Other sources of aluminum are cookware, deodorants, antacids, aluminum foils, cans and containers.

Benzoates (sodium benzoate).: Benzoic acid occurs naturally in anise, berries, black olive, blueberries, broccoli, cauliflower, cherry bark, cinnamon, cloves, cranberries, ginger, green grapes, green peas, licorice, plums, prunes, spinach, and tea. Benzoic acid or sodium benzoate is commonly used as a preservative in food processing. This is used as a flavoring agent in chocolate, orange, lemon, nut, and other flavors in beverages, baked products, candies, ice creams, and chewing gums and also used as a preservative in soft drinks, margarine, jellies, juices, pickles, and condiments.

This is also used in perfumes and cosmetics to prevent spoilage by microorganisms. Benzoic acid is a mild antifungal agent. It is metabolized by the liver. Large amount of benzoic acid or benzoates can cause intestinal disturbances, can irritate the eyes, skin, and mucous membranes. This causes eczema, acne and other skin conditions in sensitive people.

Cal. Propionate: (sodium propionate and propionic acid): These are found in dairy products, cheese, breads, cakes, baked goods and chocolate products, They are used as preservatives and mold inhibitors. They reduce the growth of molds and some bacteria.

Source: Baked products, breads, rolls, cakes, cup cakes, processed cheese, chocolate products, preserves, jellies, and butter.

Cal. Silicate: Used as an anticaking agent in products, table salt and other foods preserved in powder form used as a moisture control agent.

Carbamates: These pesticides are used widely in many places. Their toxicity is slightly lesser than some other pesticides like organochlorines. They are known to produce birth defects.

Source: pesticide-sprayed foods.

Carbon Monoxide: CO is an odorless, colorless gas that competes with oxygen for hemoglobin. The affinity of CO for hemoglobin is more than 200-fold greater than that of oxygen. CO causes tissue hypoxia. Headache is one of the first symptoms, followed by confusion, decreased visual acuity, tachycardia, syncope, metabolic acidosis, retinal hemorrhage, coma, convulsions, and death.

Source: Driving through heavy traffic, damaged gas range, leaky valves of the gas line, exhaust pipes, living in a closed up room for long time, trapped firewood smoke, smoke inhalation from being in a closed, vehicles parked, with windows closed and engine running, an automobile kept engine running in closed garage for hours, exhaust from autos and other machinery, etc.

Casein: Milk protein. Also used in prepared foods, candies, protein shakes, etc.

EDTA: This is a very efficient polydentate chelator of many divalent or trivalent cations including calcium. This is used primarily in lead poisoning. This is toxic to the kidneys. Adequate hydration is necessary when you take this in any form.

Ethylene gas (used on fruits, especially on green bananas).

Food Bleach: Most of these are used in bleaching the flour products. Benzoil peroxides, chlorine dioxides, nitrosyl chlorides, potassium bromate, mineral salts, potassium iodate, ammonium sulfate, ammonium phosphate, are the most commonly used food bleaches. They whiten the flour. They also improve the appearance. Whatever they are using should be listed on the labels but not always done. Sometimes more than one item is used for better benefit.

Formic Acid: This is a caustic, colorless, forming liquid, naturally seen in ants (ant bite), synthetically produced and used in tanning and dyeing solutions, fumigants and insecticides. This is also used as an artificial flavoring in food preparations.

Malic Acid: A colorless, highly water soluble, crystalline substance, having a pleasant sour taste, and found in apples, grapes, rhubarb, and cactus. This substance is found to be very effective in reducing general body aches. If you are allergic to it, then you can get severe body ache.

Mannan: Polysaccharides of mannose, found in various legumes and in nuts. Allergy to this factor in dried beans causes fibromyalgia-like symptoms in sensitive people.

Mannitol: It is hexahydric alcohol, used in renal function testing to measure glomerular filtration. Used intravenously as an osmotic diuretic.

Salicylic Acid: Amyl, phenyl, benzyl, and methyl salicylates).

A number of foods including almonds, apples, apricots, berries, plums, cloves, cucumbers, prunes, raisins, tomatoes, and wintergreen. Salicylic acid made synthetically by heating phenol with carbon dioxide is the basis of acetyl salicylic acid. Salicylates are also used in a variety of flavorings such as strawberry, root beer, spice, sarsaparilla, walnut, grapes, and mint.

Succinic Acid: Found in meats, cheese, fungi, and many vegetables with its distinct tart, acid taste.
Source: asparagus, broccoli, beets, and rhubarb.

Talc (magnesium silicate): Talc is a silica chalk that is used in coating, polishing rice and as an anticaking agent. It is used externally on the body surface to dry the area. Talc is thought to be carcinogenic. It may contain asbestos particles. White rice is polished and coated with it.

Tartaric Acid: This is a flavor enhancer. It is a stabilizer.
Commonly seen Water pollutants: There are many water pollutants we see in our water.
Some of them get filtered out by the time we receive in our tap. Most of these pollutants still remain in small amounts. Some of these are inorganic water pollutants like: arsenic, asbestos, cadmium, chromium, copper, cyanide, Lead, mercury, nickels, nitrates, nitrosamines, selenium, silica, silver, and zinc.

Commonly seen Water Chemicals (in drinking water).
Alum sulfate, ammonium chloride, benzene, carbon tetrachloride, chlorine, DDT, ferric chloride, gasoline, heavy metals (mercury, silver, zinc, arsenic, lead, copper), organochlorides, organophosphates, PCBs, pesticides, petroleum products, Sodium hydroxide, toluene, and xylene.

Organic chemical water pollutants: 1,2, dichloroethane, 2,4,5,T, 2,4,-D., aldicarb, benzene, carbon tetrachloride, chloroform, DDT, dibromo-chloropropane (DBCP), dichlorobenzene, dioxane, endrin, ethylene dibromide (EDB), gasoline, lindane, methoxychlor, polychlorinated biphenyls (PCB), polynuclear aromatic hydrocarbon (PAH), tetrachloroethylene, toluene, toxaphene, trichloromethane, trichloroethylene (TCE), vinyl chloride, MTBE (Methyl tertiary butyl ether is a gasoline additive), and xylene.

Some people with extreme sensitivity to these pollutants react badly with exposure by exhibiting mild to severe symptoms in various health areas. Some of the commonly seen symptoms are nausea, vomiting, diarrhea, abdominal cramps, brain fog, fatigue, body ache, joint pains, water retention in the body, flu like symptoms, fever, eczema, and rashes, sinusitis, post nasal drips, insomnia, etc. If you boil it for 30 minutes, the effect of these chemicals is reduced.

10

AUTISM CASE STUDIES

SIMON'S PROGRESSION THROUGH NAET

S imon, age nine, was diagnosed as having autism spectrum disorder with occasional seizures since the age of four. He had all the classic behaviors of autism. He was categorized as high-functional. According to his parents his autistic traits increased ten fold whenever he ate certain foods. His mother observed that his occasional seizures were connected with high consumption of refined sugar. His mother made a list of these foods: milk, eggs, wheat, bread, corn, sugar, chocolate, candy, fruits, oats, fish, beans, jelly beans, his prescription medication, hot dogs, barbecued beef, pork, chicken, brown rice, raisins, nuts, ice cream, ice cubes, potato, tomato, oranges, grapes, banana, avocado, cheese, and salsa. Certain foods made him violent and aggressive for a number of hours. He consumed enormous amounts of food which made him grow fat. He weighed 110 pounds at the age of nine. He was put on a rotation diet with a limited number of foods. It was not easy to plan his meals avoiding all of the above listed food items.

When Simon was evaluated in our office, we found the following symptoms: he avoided eye contact, played alone, showed no awareness of people, resisted physical touch by anyone including his mother, lacked appropriate social or emotional responses, lacked communication skills, was unable to talk, made unusual sounds, had extreme need for sameness, was attached to a cream colored old baby blanket, was preoccupied with twirling and pulling his hair or chewing the sleeve of his long sleeve shirt, refused to try new foods, refused to chew foods, insisted on eating fried foods and swallowed them in big chunks, was startled by any external noises, had severe insomnia, flapped his hand over his left side of the face repeatedly, showed distress and cried every now and then without any reason, wet his pants periodically, and was uncooperative in learning or doing school work. He also suffered from repeated dry skin, patches of scattered dermatitis and/or eczema, itching of his body, drooling, runny nose, canker sores, bad breath, abdominal bloating, flatulence and constipation.

He sat through the computer testing for food sensitivity screening. He was tested for 156 food items. The interpretation of the computer reading is on a scale of 0-100, (50 is normal, 100 is the maximum sensitivity at an inflammatory level, and zero is a possible hidden allergy or an artifact).

HIS EAV COMPUTER TEST RESULTS SHOWED:

148 items	100/100
6 items	96
2 items	92

Interpretation of the reading is as follows:
Severe Allergy = 90-100
Moderate to severe = 70-90
Mild to moderate = 55-70
Cellular level imbalances = 50-55
Normal = <55

NST was done through his mother using her as the surrogate. He had weakness on 20 groups of basic allergens when tested with NST. He was also found to be allergic to cotton, polyester and acrylic fabrics.

His vital signs were within normal limits. He had some scratch marks and a few scattered hives on his body. He also suffered from mild upper respiratory problems including mild dry cough (suffered for six months), itching of his nostrils, red cheeks and malar flush.

He was treated for egg mix on the first visit. On the following visit, his mother reported that he stopped coughing within hours after the first treatment (egg mix). One week after the first treatment, he still remained free of his coughing.

He was then treated for calcium mix. This included milk and milk products, calcium and vitamin D. On the following visit, his mother reported that his canker sores were healed completely. His abdominal bloating was slightly better.

Next he was treated for vitamin C mix. This included vitamin C, ascorbic acid, oxalic acid, citrus mix, vegetable mix and fruit mix. On the following visit, he appeared restless and refused to sit in the chair to wait his turn. Instead, he rushed into my office. My quick impulse was, "How are you Simon?"

"How are you Simon?" He repeated my question.

"Ah! Simon, you are speaking!" I exclaimed.

He snorted back "Ah! Simon, You are speaking!" Then his mother walked in and stood behind him with a beaming smile. I looked at his mother and said, "Wow! Did you hear him speak?" Simon immediately responded, "Wow! Did you hear him speak?"

He repeated every word I said and his mother said for the next few minutes. He also had a smile on his face all along. His mother said he was chirping away nonstop after the treatment for vitamin C. He repeated everyone's conversation throughout the week. She was so relieved to hear him speak even though his speech didn't make any sense. All these years, she never knew that he could say even one word. Now he was speaking fluently without any accent or hesitation, the words just flowed. "He did not even appear that he was listening," she said, "How could he have learned all these words and sentences without anyone teaching him I wonder!" She was still amazed at his sudden progress. Even with his strange response he had passed the treatment for vitamin C.

He was next treated for B complex, again through his mother as a surrogate. After the treatment, he was asked to sit outside along with his mother with the sample placed inside his sock. In a few minutes he got up from his seat, rushed into my office and fell on the treatment table. Another patient was sitting at the same table discussing her treatment plan with me. I looked at his face. His cheeks and ears were turning red. He was burning with fever (103 degree Farenheit by axilla) . I immediately took the sample of B vitamins out of his sock, called his mother in and repeated NAET and in a few minutes the redness of his cheeks and ears diminished and his temperature started coming down. I made him rest in one of the treatment rooms along with his mother, periodically checking his condition. He rested quietly dozing on and off. I repeated NAET treatment three more times every 15 minutes for the B complex during the next hour. It took about an hour to get his temperature down to normal. He became very quiet and appeared tired. After he became stable, his mother took him home.

On the following visit, Simon sat quietly in his seat. He did not jump around or move from his seat this time. His mother said he was extremely quiet after the B complex treatment. He did not talk but nodded his head for all the questions appropriately by "yes" or "no." She said he looked as if he had no energy to say a word. But when I checked him he had passed the treatment for B complex with flying colors.

He was treated for sugar mix next. In less than a few minutes, he broke out in hives all over his body. NAET was repeated immediately on him through a surrogate (his mother). We repeated NAET every five minutes for six times until he passed the sugar mix. His hives faded away in just a few minutes and he fell asleep. His mother had to carry him to the car since he refused to wake up. He seemed to be having a very restful sleep.

On the following visit, he looked cheerful, quiet, calm, and appeared shy. He wouldn't look at other patients and he used his mother's body as a shield to hide behind her. He covered his face with his hands and peeked through his finger-gaps. But he kept smiling all along. His mother said she had not noticed this kind of behavior before.

He was treated for iron mix that day. Soon after the iron treatment, there was a sudden change in his calm disposition. In a few minutes, he became very aggressive. He began kicking his mother, tried to push her out of the chair, and his smiling face was replaced by an angry and unhappy one. Then he began to bang his head on the wall and scream.

He wouldn't cooperate to walk to the treatment room. He crawled his way to the corner then went under the treatment table in the acupuncture room and hid there like a frightened kitten. He refused to come out. We had to move the table physically to get him out of there. We had to carry him to the NAET treatment room. NAET was repeated through the surrogate every five minutes for four more times. By then, he calmed down. His calmness projected as deep sleep. He curled up into a fetal position. By then we were familiar with his response. After the 20 minute waiting period from the last NAET treatment, his mother carried him to the car.

On the next visit, his mother said he had slept for 18 hours without eating, drinking, or moving from his fetal position. When he woke up he looked tired. He was too tired to eat anything. His mother fed him. He ate slowly and calmly.

Then he went to sleep again. He slept for three days intermittently for hours. He was not interested in any activities. So his mother let him sleep. After three days when he woke up, he was his usual self again. But he was less aggressive and behaved somewhat normally. He pointed to certain foods like ice creams, cookies, etc., indicating that he wanted to eat them, which he had never done before. His mother let him have the cookies and ice cream since he was treated and cleared for sugar and milk.

On the following visit, he came and sat down on the chair in the waiting room. He had a serious look on his face.

Kevin, another seven-year-old normal patient, was demanding that his mother take him to Burger King. Simon watched him for a while and stood up from his chair pointing his index finger towards Kevin and told him in a firm voice, "You are naughty!" Everyone in the waiting room laughed and complemented him saying, "Very good, Simon!" He smiled. He began to develop appropriate responses.

He was treated for vitamin A mix next. This included fish, shellfish, beta carotene and fish oils. In a few minutes after the treatment, he began itching all over his body. He was treated two more times for vitamin A, every five minutes and his itching stopped. Compared to all other previous treatments, the vitamin A treatment seemed easy. He fell asleep again demonstrating that his brain and body were happy to have another culprit out of his body.

On the next visit, his mother was beaming with joy. She said Simon's skin felt very soft and all the eczema and dermatitis cleared up. He stopped scratching his body. His dry scalp also cleared up. He was treated for mineral mix.

Once again, he became very aggressive in the office. I had to treat him five times every five minutes to make his brain accept the mineral mix. After the treatment, he fell asleep again and his mother had to carry him to the car.

On the following visit, he seemed to be full of energy. When the car stopped in the parking lot, he ran ahead of his mother into the office, ran to my assistant who was standing in the front office, hugged her and kissed her hand. Then without a word, he ran into my office, and hugged me, looked into my eyes and said: "I love you, Dr. Devi."

His mother waited impatiently to see what would happen when he completed all the allergens in the NAET Basic set. We had to do one at a time on each session, sometimes, each one needed to be repeated a few times before his body could release the allergic bond. After completing all the basic allergens, he was treated for serotonin, dopamine, neurotransmitters, secretin, dimethyl glycine, tap water, amino acids, starch complex, alcohol, caffeine, chocolate, food colors, food additives, stomach acids, digestive enzymes, parasite mix, childhood immunization (MMR, DPT, Polio), his past and present medications, pesticides, fabrics, plastics, latex, and chemicals. He was also treated for all the animals and toys in his house. Soon after the treatment for vaccinations, his seizures stopped. We repeated the computer test several times. The final test showed 10 reading between 50 and 55 and nothing above 55.

He is a healthy teenager now who can eat any food of his choice without any adverse reaction. He is attending a regular school and living a normal life now.

SPENCER'S JOURNEY THROUGH NAET

Treated by Jackie Smiley, N.D., Riverside, CA

Spencer was 4-years-old at the time of his first visit. His mother said that he was developing normally until his 18-month booster shot. Following the shot he ran a fever for three days, slept for 18 hours, and would spend his time staring at the TV. In public he would scream. He came into the office with a bag of potato chips. His mother said that was all he would eat and insisted on always taking them with him. He was treated for the potato chips first, and Spencer immediately lost his craving for them. Within two treatments he was able to give them up and began to eat better food.

He was treated for: frontal and temporal lobes, B complex, potato chips and B complex, sugars, TB, smallpox, measles, chicken pox and mumps vaccines. At this point his speech therapy teacher said he was interacting more, and speaking with three words. He was involved with other children for the first time.

Spencer was then treated for minerals, Vitamin A, French-fries, fats-repeated one time, DPT—repeated one time and Pertussis—repeated one time. After these treatments Spencer was asking questions like, "What's in there?"

At this point, Oct. 31, 1996, Spencer took a 5-month break from his sessions. During this time he stopped making the expected progress in his therapy classes. It was apparent that the sessions not only helped him with allergens but also balanced his energy so he could be more receptive to learning.

His mother stated, "Every time Spencer stops his NAET treatments, he stops progressing in other areas of his life."

RESUMING IN APRIL, SPENCER WAS TREATED FOR:

Amino acids
Salts and Chlorides
Artificial Sweeteners
Potatoes
Hong Kong Flu
Food colors and Additives
Flax seed oil
Tetracycline
Doughnuts—repeated
Wheat+ Yeast+ Sugar
Wheat+ Milk mix+ Sugar
Udo's oil
Vit. E
Vit. F
(Vit. K & D were good)

By this time, Spencer was making such developmental progress that he was signed up for public schooling for the fall semester.

Next we treated him for:
Herpes virus
Food Color and Serotonin
Chemicals
Vit. T
Red Candy
Candida & Mercury
Eggs & Chicken

Opioids
Virus & Brain
Calcium

His mother summarized Spencer's NAET experience by saying, "It was so beneficial and natural. He can talk, focus and learn. To be able to do this naturally, without drugs or dietary changes is tremendous. He eliminated his allergies to the environment and food with NAET. He never needed a casein or gluten free diet."

NAET DAYS OF DYLAN O

Dylan O. was five-years-old when he began NAET. He suffered from ADD and PDD/ mild autism. Along with this he exhibited angry behavior. He had been expelled from four preschools. His diet was almost totally sugar based, and he craved sugar and doughnuts.

His sessions followed the standard order. After the Basics we treated him for doughnuts. It took five treatments for him to clear them. After thirteen treatments his behavior has greatly improved. He then got good reports from his teachers, craved less sugar and was off Ritalin.

FOOD- INDUCED AUTISM

Clayton, age 9, had food-induced autism. He tested very well and had no autistic traits whatsoever unless he ate certain foods. If his mother gave him a hot dog before testing he behaved severely autistic. In addition to autism, he exhibited violent/psychotic behavior. He had been placed on anti-psychotic medication to curb the violence, which had helped for a time, however, he was beginning to break through the medication. For example he chased his younger sister around the house with a knife. His parents knew if they couldn't calm him down, he would have to be placed in another home in order to protect their daughter.

While Clayton's mother was pregnant with him, their neighborhood was sprayed with Malathion. While eight months pregnant she had intrauterine seizures. At birth, Clayton's blood sugar level dropped. At one-month-old he had pneumonia and was placed on antibiotics. The mother noticed quite a difference in him after this. He was lethargic, would cry a lot, scream and stiffen his body.

We followed the Basics beginning with eggs/chicken. After the Basics we did diphtheria, tetanus, pneumonia, and fruit mix. Clayton's violence abated and he was able to go off anti-psychotic medication. His mother was so relieved that he could remain at home. At this point she got a job and was unable to bring him in. In only 10 treatments he made significant progress. Further treatments would greatly enhance his well being. We have yet to treat him for hot dogs, for example.

DRUG- INDUCED AUTISM

Christian, age 2 ¾ was born addicted to Methadone and, most likely, other drugs as well. He was in drug withdrawal for the first three months of life. A foster family had raised him his entire life as his mother was in jail. In addition to ADD he was very violent. He was unable to play with other children because he would harm them. His physician had placed him on Risperedol for his aggression but it wasn't helpful. As a matter of fact, most drugs were useless for him. The week before his first NAET treatment his neurologist told his foster mother, "Sometimes with these drug addicted children it just doesn't work out and they need to be institutionalized."

On the first visit to my office he punched and kicked his foster mother and foster sisters. He screamed the entire time as well. He did all of this while on 12 mg. of Ritalin. In just one treatment of egg/chicken he was able to go off the Ritalin.

Here is an account of the progress he made, according to his foster mother:

Egg mix/chicken: No Ritalin for 25 hours

Calcium mix/Milk mix: He was normal, quiet but still failed the treatment.

Calcium mix/Milk mix: He is a kid instead of a frustrating kid. He sat in a grocery cart one whole hour for the first time.

Infant formula—At nearly three-years-old, he would live on formula and didn't like food. He tested very allergic to the formula. We had to treat him emotionally for the formula as well.

Vitamin C mix (Bioflavonoid/Citrus)

B Complex/Wheat, Gluten: slept two nights, very unusual. His behavior has been awful since then. He was tested for Dimetapp. This was causing his hyperactive behavior. He had to be treated for Dimetapp and combinations:

Dimetapp/Tryptophane, Dimetapp/Brain

Vitamin A mix /Fish, shellfish mix: No screaming, but constant movement

Mineral Mix: Nothing unusual

Salt mix, Chlorides: Treatment not needed

Grain mix: No treatment

Stomach Acids: Nothing unusual.

Macaroni

Stomach

Stomach/Enzymes/Secretin/Sugar enzymes

Candida

Candida/Brain

Candida/Heavy Metals/Mercury

Virus mix

Food color/ Food additives

Food color and food additives/adrenals

Food color and additives/sugar

Cocaine-made symptoms worse

Marijuana—was real calm for a day, then awful

Marijuana—the second treatment calmed him down again

Methadone, Methadone/Hormones

LSD

Bacteria mix

Bacteria/Eustachian tubes/Ear mix/Cochlea

String cheese

String cheese/Thymus/Lymph.

Pollen mix: failed the first time

Pollen mix
Pollen/mountain pollen/ local pollen
Otter Pops
Weeds/Pigweed/Local weeds
Spice mix 1/Spice mix 2

Christian was then able to go without medication, didn't scream or hit. He was such a different child that his other treating doctors were amazed

Jacqueline Smillie, ND
NAET Specialist
Redlands, CA

AUTISM AND PDD

NAET Practitioner: Glenn Nozek, D.C., Toms River, NJ.

Stephen S. was diagnosed as autistic when he was four-years-old. His family heard about NAET in March 1998 when he was nine years of age. NAET treatments were started on March 19, 1998, when he was treated for egg mix.

March 23: Calcium mix. For 15 minutes after the NAET treatment for calcium, his left ear turned red and hot.

March 26: Calcium mix was repeated.

For 15 minutes after treatment, his left ear turned red and hot. After this treatment, his teacher wrote a note and stated, "Stephen's behavior is exceptional. I don't know if you are doing anything different, we are not. He seems to really enjoy learning now and he is understanding directions which lessens his frustrations." I also note an increase in receptive language. He will now answer most questions by nodding his head yes or no. He also is more aware of everything.

On March 28th, he played outside appropriately all day (Stephen usually chooses to stay indoors watching TV). He was running and kicking and throwing a ball. He had appropriate interactions with a neighbor boy and his sister.

March 30: He was tested for vitamin C (found negative). Then I tested him and treated for B complex. For 15 minutes his ears were red and hot. He developed hives on his face and a few on his torso. A note came from his speech therapist the next day stating that "his receptive language/vocabulary has grown incredibly high. He understands everything!"

April 2: Vitamin B complex repeated with RNA and DNA.

During the 15 minutes after treatment, his ears were red and hot. Hives appeared around his eyes and his eyelids reddened. A few hives were seen on the torso, which subsided after 10 minutes.

Stephen's other basic NAET treatments passed without any significant reactions. He is a normal child now.

Glen Nozek, D.C.
Toms River, NJ

11

NUTRITION CORNER

Many people take vitamin and mineral supplements nowadays. The quality of the food is far worse than years ago. The food products we buy in the market have less food value than necessary, so it has become a necessity to supplement our food if we are to prevent malnutrition.

Vitamins and trace minerals are essential to life. Vitamins are compounds required for biochemical reactions, which cannot be synthesized in higher animals but must be obtained in diet. Vitamins are generally classified in two categories. Water soluble (B vitamins, folate, biotin, pantothenate) are stored very little and have to be supplied frequently. Fat soluble vitamins (vitamin A, D, E, K) can be stored in tissue and thus pose a risk for toxicity when taken in excess. Vitamins are precursors of cofactors in numerous chemical reactions in the body. Examples of some functions are:

B vitamins are used in enzymatic functions.

Vitamin A is involved in the visual processes and regulation of transcription.

Vitamin C and E are used in reducing reactions

Vitamin K is necessary in the coagulation of blood, etc.

Vitamin D is important in bone formation and for absorption of calcium in the body.

It is formed by the body when the skin is exposed to sunlight (ultraviolet light).

For those who avoid exposure to sunlight and for black people who are protected from ultraviolet light by skin pigment, vitamin D fortified milk or a vitamin D supplement may be necessary. They contribute to good health by regulating the metabolism and assisting the biochemical processes that release energy from the foods and drinks we consume. Vitamins and trace minerals are micronutrients, and the body needs them in small amounts. The lack of these essential elements even though they are needed in minute amounts can create various impairments and tissue damage in the body.

Water, carbohydrates, fats, proteins and bulk minerals like calcium, magnesium, sodium, potassium and phosphorus are considered to be macronutrients, taken into the body via regular food. They are needed in larger amounts. Both macro- and micronutrients are not only necessary to produce energy for our daily bodily functions, but also for growth and development of the body and mind.

Using macronutrients (food & drinks) and micronutrients (vitamins and trace minerals), the body creates some essential chemicals, enzymes and hormones. These are the foundations of human bodily functions. Enzymes are the catalysts or simple activators in the chemical reactions that are continually taking place in the body. Without the appropriate vitamins and trace minerals, the production and functions of the enzymes will be incomplete. Prolonged deficiency of these vitamins and minerals can produce immature or incomplete enzyme production, protein synthesis, cell mutation, immature RNA, DNA synthesis, etc., which can mimic various organic diseases in the body.

Deficiency of vitamins and other essentials in the body can be due to poor intake and absorption.

Many autistic children and adults have nutritional deficiencies due to poor eating habits and will benefit from nutritional supplements and megavitamin therapy. Others may have nutritional deficiencies due to food allergies and will not show any improvements on vitamin therapy.

All autistic people should be tested for possible allergies. If they are found to be allergic, they should be treated for the allergies before they are supplemented with vitamins and minerals.

When a patient is allergic to vitamin B complex, in many cases he/she cannot digest grains, resulting in B complex deficiencies. When one gets treated for allergies via NAET, he/she can eat grains, without any ill effect and will begin to assimilate B complex vitamins. In some cases through NTP, I have found B complex deficiency amounting to fifteen to twenty times the normal daily-recommended allowances. After supplementing with large amounts of B complex for a few weeks (10 – 20 times RDA amount per day for a week or so), the deficiency was eliminated. Over and over in hundreds of patients, after supplementing for weeks, we have been able to remove their vitamin B complex deficiency symptoms completely. This proves that even though water soluble, vitamin B complex is still stored in the body. We have received similar results with vitamin C. But more research is needed on a larger number of patients to verify these findings.

Fat-soluble vitamins are stored for longer periods of time in the body's fatty tissues and the liver. When you are allergic to fat soluble vitamins, you begin to store them in unwanted places of the body. Some of the abnormal fat-soluble vitamin storage can be seen as lipomas, warts, skin tags, benign tumors inside or outside the body, etc.

Taking vitamins and minerals in their proper balance is important for the correct functioning of all vitamins. Excess consumption of an isolated vitamin or mineral can produce unpleasant symptoms of that particular nutrient. High doses of one element can also cause depletion of other nutrients in the body, leading to other problems. Most of these vitamins work synergistically, complementing and/or strengthening each other's function.

Vitamins and minerals should be taken with meals unless specified otherwise. Oil-soluble vitamins should be taken before meals, and water-soluble vitamins should be taken between or after meals. But when you are taking megadoses of any of these, they should always be taken with or after meals. Vitamins and minerals, as nutritional supplements taken with meals, will supply the missing nutrients in our daily diets.

Synthetic vitamins are produced in a laboratory from isolated chemicals with similar characteristics to natural vitamins. Although there are no major chemical differences between a vitamin found in food and one created in a laboratory, natural supplements do not contain other unnatural ingredients. Supplements that are not labeled natural may include coal tars, artificial coloring, preservatives, sugars, and starches, as well as other binding agents and additives. Vitamins labeled natural may not contain vitamins that have not been extracted from a natural food source. One must select carefully.

There are various books available on nutrition today that are helpful in understanding vitamins and their assimilative processes. If you are interested in learning more about nutrition, if you do not get enough understanding about vitamins and other nutritional supplements from this concise chapter, you are advised to read the appropriate book titles listed in the bibliography section at the end of this book.

VITAMIN A

Clinical studies have proven vitamin A and beta-carotene to be very powerful immune-stimulants and protective agents.

Vitamin A is necessary for proper vision and in preventing night blindness, skin disorders, and acne. It protects the body against colds, influenza and other infections. It enhances immunity, helps heal ulcers and wounds and maintains the epithelial cell tissue. It is necessary for the growth of bones and teeth.

Vitamin A works best with B complex, vitamin D, vitamin E, calcium, phosphorus and zinc. Zinc is needed to get vitamin A out of the liver, where it is usually stored. Large doses of vitamin A should be taken only under proper supervision, because it can accumulate in the body and become toxic.

Many teenagers with an allergy to vitamin A have acne, blemishes and other skin problems. People with allergy to vitamin A develop skin tags, and warts, and pimples around the neck, arms, etc. It causes retention of water in the tissue resulting in premenstrual syndrome. When they get treated and properly supplemented with vitamin A, the skin clears up and PMS problems become less severe.

VITAMIN D

Vitamin D is often called the sunshine vitamin. It is a fat-soluble vitamin, acquired through sunlight or food sources. Vitamin D is absorbed from foods, through the intestinal wall, after they are ingested. Smog reduces the vitamin D producing rays of the sun. Dark-skinned people and sun-tanned people do not absorb vitamin D from the sun. Vitamin D helps the utilization of calcium and phosphorus in the human body. When there is an allergy to vitamin D, the vitamin is not absorbed into the body through foods, or from the sun. People with an allergy to vitamin D can exhibit deficiency syndromes: rickets, severe tooth decay, softening of teeth and bones, osteomalacia, osteoporosis, sores on the skin, blisters on the skin while walking in the sun, severe sunburns when exposed to the sun, etc. Sometimes allergic persons can show toxic symptoms if they take vitamin D without clearing its allergy. These symptoms include mental confusion, unusual thirst, sore eyes, itching skin, vomiting, diarrhea, urinary urgency, calcium deposits in the blood vessels and bones, restlessness in the sun, inability to bear heat, sun radiation, electrical radiation, emotional imbalance like depression, suicidal thoughts in the winter when the sunlight is diminished. Some people in Alaska and other cold countries suffer emotional instabilities during winter (Seasonal affective Disorders or SAD) where they have a few hours of daylight in winter. When they get treated for vitamin D, and combinations, with NAET, they do not suffer from depression anymore. From this experience, it should be assumed that vitamin D is very necessary to maintain mental stability. Vitamin D works best with vitamin A, vitamin C, choline, calcium, and phosphorus.

VITAMIN E

Vitamin E is an antioxidant. The body needs zinc in order to maintain the proper levels of vitamin E in the blood. Vitamin E is a fat-soluble vitamin and is stored in the liver, fatty tissues, heart, muscles, testes, uterus, blood, adrenal and pituitary glands. Vitamin E is excreted in the feces if too much is taken.

VITAMIN K

Vitamin K is needed for blood clotting and bone formation. Vitamin K is necessary to convert glucose into glycogen for storage in the liver. Vitamin K is a fat-soluble vitamin, very essential to the formation of prothrombin, a blood-clotting material. It helps in the blood-clotting mechanism, prevents hemorrhages (nosebleeds and intestinal bleeding) and helps reduce excessive menstrual flow.

An allergy to vitamin K can produce deficiency syndromes such as prolonged bleeding time, intestinal diseases like sprue, etc., and colitis.

VITAMIN B

Approximately 15 vitamins make up the B complex family. Each one of them has unique, very important functions in the body. If the body does not absorb and utilize any or all of the B-vitamins, various health problems can result. B complex vitamins are very essential for emotional, physical and physiological well being of the human body. It is a nerve food, so it is necessary for the proper growth and maintenance of the nervous system and brain function. It also keeps the nerves well fed so that nerves are kept calm and the autistic person can maintain a good mental attitude.

B-vitamins are seen in almost all foods we eat. Cooking and heating destroy some of them, others are not destroyed by processing or preparation. People who are allergic to B-vitamins can get mild to severe reactions just by eating the foods alone. If they are supplemented with vitamin B complex, without being aware of the allergies, such people can get exaggerated reactions. One has to be very cautious when taking B complex, commonly called stress vitamins.

Dr. Carlton Frederic, in his book, "Psychonutrition," tried to point out that nutritional deficiencies are the causes of most of the mental irritations such as extreme anger, severe mood swings, bipolar diseases, schizophrenic disorders, frontal lobe disorders, anxiety disorders, attention deficit disorders, hyperactivity disorders, various neurological disorders, mental sicknesses including mild to moderate to severe psychiatric disorders. He tried to prove his theory by giving large doses of vitamin B complex, especially B-12, to some of the psychiatric patients. Fifty percent of the patients got better, were cured of their mental sickness and went back to live normal lives. But another 50 percent made no progress or got worse. He couldn't explain why the other 50% got worse. His theory was ridiculed and his treatment protocol with mega B complex vitamin therapy for mental disorders was thrown out for want of proof. He did not think in the direction of allergies. When I discovered the allergic connection, I tried to contact him to let him know that his theory was absolutely right and I had proof to support his theory. Unfortunately, I was a year late to reach him. He had passed away a year before my discovery of NAET.

A few minerals are extremely essential for our daily functions. While some metals and trace minerals are mentioned here, for more information on other minerals, please refer to the appropriate references in the bibliography.

CALCIUM

Calcium is one of the essential minerals in the body. Calcium works with phosphorus, magnesium, iron, vitamins A, C and D. Calcium helps to maintain strong bones and healthy teeth. It regulates the heart functions and helps to relax the nerves and muscles. It induces relaxation and sleep.

Deficiencies in calcium can result in rickets, osteomalacia, osteoporosis, hyperactivity, restlessness, inability to relax, generalized aches and pains, joint pains, formation of bone spurs, backaches, PMS, cramps in the legs and heavy menstrual flow.

Many autistic children and adults respond well to calcium supplementation. Often autistic people suffer from abdominal pains, dysentery, insomnia, skin problems, nervousness, dyslexia, canker sores, post-nasal drip, hyperactivity, obesity, and joint disorders. They all respond well to calcium supplementation after allergy elimination. When people are on cortisone treatment, they need to take more calcium.

IRON

Poor diet is certainly one cause of iron deficiency but if you are allergic to iron, you do not absorb iron. Iron is absorbed better in the acid medium (stomach) but in the intestine where the digestive juices are basic, iron does not absorb well. If you have a deficiency of iron, or if you have an allergy to iron and base in combination, all iron containing food can cause bloating and abdominal distention. Iron deficiency results in anemia. If you have an iron deficiency you can get various health problems. If you are allergic to iron, and if you supplement with iron or eat iron-containing foods, you may experience various allergic reactions like dry mouth, fatigue, dizziness, nausea, loss of appetite, restlessness, a short attention span, feeling extreme cold, cold limbs, internal cold and tremors, cold extremities, feels better in warm weather, poor circulation in the fingers and toes, varicose veins and fragile arteries, hair loss, insomnia, swelling of the feet and ankles, etc. Iron deficiency also can give rise to above symptoms. Iron is also necessary to maintain the health of blood cells especially red blood cells. This improves the absorption of oxygen and elimination of carbon dioxide and other toxins from blood. Iron plays an important role in awareness and alertness. An imbalance of iron in the blood causes sluggish synaptic functions in the nerve endings causing the neuro-transmitters to function poorly resulting in behavior and learning disability in young children. So good assimilation and utilization of iron is necessary for body's natural detoxification and maintenance function. Vitamin C can enhance the iron absorption. A high fiber diet, and the repeated daily use of laxatives can deplete iron from your body. Drinking tea can deplete iron in the body. Drinking tea (tannic acid) with meals can inhibit the iron absorption from food.

Food sources: chicken liver, beef liver, beef, crab, soybean, blackstrap molasses, spinach, beets, beet green, beef, potato, scallops, sunflower seeds, pistachio, broccoli, cashew nuts, lima beans, Swiss chard, turkey dark-meat, lobster, tuna, almonds, sesame seeds, peanuts, peas, prunes, apricot, Brussels sprouts, cod, raisins, haddock, and endive.

CHROMIUM

Chromium is a natural insulin regulator. It is essential for insulin to work efficiently in our bodies. Insulin is required to remove glucose (sugar) from the blood. Chromium helps the insulin to do its job so that blood sugar can be kept at a normal range.

Food sources: sugar, whole grains, wheat germ, corn, corn oil, brewers yeast, mushrooms, red meat, liver, shellfish, clams and chicken.

COBALT

Cobalt is essential to form quality red blood cells, since it is part of vitamin B-12. Deficiency results in B-12 anemia. Multiple chemically sensitive people have low tolerance to any external smells like gasoline, smoke, chemical fumes, sprays, perfumes, etc. Maintaining a good level of cobalt along with selenium and molybdenum helps to reduce the smell-sensitivity in MCS people. If they are allergic to any of the trio, they should be treated singly or in combination before supplementation.

Food sources: green leafy vegetables, milk, buckwheat, figs, red meat, liver, kidney, oyster, and clams.

COPPER

Copper is required to convert the body's iron into hemoglobin. Combined with the thyroxin, it helps to produce the pigment factor for hair and skin. It is essential for utilization of vitamin C. Deficiency results in anemia and edema. Toxicity symptoms and allergic symptoms are insomnia, hair loss, irregular menses, joint pains, arthritis and depression.

Food sources: almonds, green beans, peas, green leafy vegetables, whole wheat, other whole grains, dried beans, prunes, raisins, beef-liver, shellfish, and fish.

FLUORIDE

Sodium fluoride is often added to drinking water. Calcium fluoride is seen in natural food sources. Fluorine decreases chances of dental carries, (too much can discolor teeth). It also strengthens the bones. Deficiency leads to tooth decay. Toxicity and allergy symptoms include dizziness, nausea, vomiting, fatigue, poor appetite, skin rashes, itching, yeast infections, mental confusion, muscle spasms, mental fogginess and arthritis. Treatment for fluoride will eliminate possible allergies.

Food sources: fluoridated water, gelatin, sunflower seeds, milk, cheese, carrots, almonds, green leafy vegetables and fish.

IODINE

Two thirds of the body's iodine is in the body's thyroid gland. Since the thyroid gland controls metabolism, and iodine influences the thyroid, an under supply of this mineral can result in weight gain, general fatigue and slow mental reaction. Iodine helps to keep the body thin, promotes growth, gives more energy, improves mental alertness, and promotes the growth of hair, nails and teeth. Autistic children are found to be allergic to iodine, causing poor absorption of the substance. Some autistic children crave salt. They may not be receiving sufficient iodine in their diet or may have poor absorption of iodine due to an allergy. A deficiency in iodine can cause overweight, hypothyroidism, goiter and lack of energy.

Food sources: kelp, seafood, iodized salt, vegetables grown in iodine-rich soil, and onion.

MAGNESIUM

This is one of the important minerals to help with irritability and hyperactivity. Magnesium is necessary for the metabolism of calcium, vitamin C, phosphorus, sodium, potassium and vitamin A. It is essential for the normal functioning of nerves and muscles. Autistic and hyperactive children need more magnesium in their diet to maintain the stability of the nervous system. It also helps convert blood sugar into energy. It works as a natural tranquilizer, laxative and diuretic. Diuretics deplete magnesium. Alcoholics and asthmatics are deficient in magnesium.

Food sources: Nuts, soybean, green leafy vegetables, almonds, brown rice, whole grains, sesame seeds and sunflower seeds.

MANGANESE

Manganese helps to activate digestive enzymes in the body. It is important in the formation of thyroxin, the principal hormone of the thyroid gland. It is necessary for the proper digestion and utilization of food. Manganese is important in reproduction and the normal functioning of the central nervous system. It helps to eliminate fatigue, improves memory, reduces nervous irritability and relaxes the mind. A deficiency may result in recurrent attacks of dizziness and poor memory.

Food sources: green leafy vegetables, beets, blueberries, oranges, grapefruit, apricot, the outer coating of nuts, and grains, peas, kelp, raw egg yolk, nuts and wheat germ.

MOLYBDENUM

Molybdenum helps in carbohydrate and fat metabolism. It is a vital part of the enzyme responsible for iron utilization. It also helps reduce allergic reaction to smell in chemically sensitive people in combination with selenium and cobalt.

Food sources: whole grains, brown rice, brewers yeast, legumes, buckwheat, millet, and dark green leafy vegetables.

PHOSPHORUS

Phosphorus is involved in virtually all physiological chemical reactions in the body. It is necessary for normal bone and teeth formation. It is important for heart regularity, and is essential for normal kidney function. It provides energy and vigor by helping in the fat and carbohydrate metabolism. It promotes growth and repairs in the body. It is essential for healthy gums and teeth. Vitamin D and calcium are essential for its proper functioning.

Food sources: whole grains, seeds, nuts, legumes, egg yolk, fish, corn, dried fruits, milk, cheese, yogurt, chicken, turkey and red meat.

POTASSIUM

Potassium works with sodium to regulate the body's water balance and to regulate the heart rhythm. It helps in clear thinking by sending oxygen to the brain. A deficiency in potassium results in edema, hypoglycemia, nervous irritability, and muscle weakness.

Food sources: vegetables, orange, banana, cantaloupe, tomatoes, mint leaves, water cress, potatoes, whole grains, seeds, nuts and cream of tartar.

SELENIUM

Selenium is an antioxidant. It works with vitamin E, slowing down the aging process. It prevents hardening of tissues and helps to retain youthful appearance. Selenium is also known to alleviate hot flashes and menopausal distress. It prevents dandruff. Some researchers have found selenium to neutralize certain carcinogens and provide protection from some cancers. It has been also found to reduce the sensitivity to smells and odors from plastics, formaldehyde, perfume, molds, smoke, and gasoline etc. It works when combined with cobalt and molybdenum.

Food sources: brewers yeast, wheat germ, kelp, sea water, sea salt, garlic, mushrooms, seafood, milk, eggs, whole grains, beef, dried beans, bran, onions, tomato and broccoli.

SODIUM

Sodium is essential for normal growth and normal body functioning. It works with potassium to maintain the sodium-potassium pump in the body. Potassium is found inside the cells and sodium is found outside.

Food sources: kelp, celery, romaine lettuce, watermelon, seafood, processed foods with salt, fast foods, table salt, fish, shellfish, carrots, beets, artichoke, dried beef, cured meats, bacon, ham, brain, kidney, watercress, sea weed, oats, avocado, Swiss chard, tomatoes, cabbage, cucumber, asparagus, pineapple, tap water, canned or frozen foods.

SULFUR

Sulfur is essential for healthy hair, skin and nails. It helps maintain the oxygen balance necessary for proper brain function. It works with B-complex vitamins for basic body metabolism. It is a part of tissue building amino acid. It tones up the skin and makes the hair lustrous and helps fight bacterial infection.

Food sources: radish, turnip, onion, celery, string beans, watercress, soybean, fish, meat, dried beans, eggs and cabbage.

VANADIUM

Vanadium prevents heart attacks. It inhibits the formation of cholesterol in blood vessels. It also regulates sugar metabolism.

Food sources: fish, seaweed, seafood.

ZINC

Zinc is essential to form certain enzymes and hormones in the body. It is very necessary for protein synthesis. It is important for blood stability and in maintaining the body's acid-alkaline balance. It is important in the development of reproductive organs and helps to normalize the prostate glands in males. It helps in treatment of mental disorders and speeds up healing of wounds and cuts on the body. Zinc helps with the growth of fingernails and eliminates cholesterol deposits in the blood vessels. It helps to improve the immune system.

Food sources: wheat bran, wheat germ, seeds, dried beans, peas, onions, mushrooms, brewers yeast, milk, eggs, oysters, herring, brown rice, fish, lamb, beef, pork, and green leafy vegetables.

TRACE MINERALS

Even though trace minerals are needed in our body, they are seen in trace amounts only. The researchers do not know definite functions of the trace minerals but deficiencies can definitely contribute toward health problems.

PROTEINS

Proteins, from the Greek *proteios*, meaning first, are a class of organic compounds which are present in and vital to every living cell. In the form of skin, hair, nails, cartilage, muscles, tendons and ligaments, proteins hold together, protect, and provide structure to the body of a multicelled organism. In the form of enzymes, hormones, antibodies, and globulins, they catalyze, regulate, and protect the body chemistry. In the form of hemoglobin, myoglobin and various lipoproteins, they effect the transport of oxygen and other substances within an organism.

Even though there are many amino acids, twenty-two of them are vital to carry out most of the functions listed above. Amino acids are essential for normal body function, from transmission of the genetic information to the growth and maintenance of the cells of the individual organism. Body cells are able to build their own proteins from amino acids, and carry out many essential functions by means of proteins. Proteins also serve as energy sources under certain situations.

Some of the researchers work with biochemistry and nutrition strongly believe and try to support their claims by various studies that most of the human illnesses we see are arising from nutritional deficiencies due to poor intake, poor digestion and malabsorption of proteins. Overconsumption of refined carbohydrates, saturated fats, poor intake of proteins cause to have lower immune system. Some researchers have predicted that one out of two Americans will die from the effects of cardiovascular disease (CVD). One out of four Americans will die from cancer. Immune deficiency disorders are sky-rocketting. Every second person we see suffer from either fibromyalgia or chronic fatigue syndrome. There are many studies performed on inborn errors of protein metabolism. It is the ignorance of human nutritional needs that will cause the overwhelming majority of Americans to suffer and become the victims of these afflictions. But it is sad to note that none of these researchers have any clue why so many people are suffering from this many nutritional disorders. No one thinks the reason for poor digestion, poor absorption or utilization of the nutrients are due to simple food allergies. When the allergies are removed with NAET, our patients begin to digest, absorb and assimilate nutrition from their daily diet and we see significant improvement in all of the above health disorders. Proteins have various functions in the body. Commonly known body function with proteins are given below:

Proteins make the skin elastic, flexible and tough.
Hair and nails are made from proteins.
Muscles, tendons, ligaments, bone matrix and joints surfaces are made from proteins.
Retina of the eye, vitreous fluid, and lenses of the eyes are made from proteins.
Blood vessels, nerves, lymphatic vessels are made from proteins.
Immune cells, body secretions like hormones, semen, mucus, are made from proteins.

PROTEINS CAN BE CLASSIFIED ON THE BASIS OF THEIR PHYSIOLOGICAL FUNCTIONS.

1. Enzymes, which catalyze body processes.

2. Hormones, which regulate body processes.

3. Formation of antibodies to protect the body.

4. Structural proteins, which constitute cartilage, skin, nails, and hair.

5. Contractile proteins, which make up the skeletal muscle.

6. Blood proteins such as hemoglobin and albumin.

FOOD SOURCE

The only complete food source for all of the amino acids used by the body is red meat (beef, meat, fish, chicken, egg) fowl and seafood. Other foods that contain a fair amount of protein: cottage cheese, any cheese, dried beans, whole grains, yogurt, milk, almond, gelatin, nuts, broccoli, brown rice, tofu, enriched bread.

DIGESTION, ABSORPTION AND UTILIZATION

Protein digestion will start from the stomach. Enzyme hydrochloric acid, gastrin, pepsin, etc. will work on it to denature the protein. Main digestion takes place in the small intestine. From the lumen of the small intestine, amino acids are transported to the mucosa cells. The body's access to amino acid is regulated by the liver. If there is any disturbance in the function anywhere in the processing and transport system, it prevents utilization of the nutrients. So one needs to check for any obstruction in the pathway.

Dietary amino acids are classified as "essential" or "non-essential." Essential amino acids (threonine, isoleucine,

leucine, valine, Iysine, methionine, phenylalanine, histidine and tryptophan) cannot be manufactured by the body and must be supplied in the diet or ill-health results. The non-essential amino acids are also essential for health but can be synthesized in the body from the essential amino acids. Both the essential and non-essential amino acids are reassembled as hormones, enzymes, neurotransmitters (chemical messengers), antibodies and nutrient carriers. A diet without any one of them will eventually cause disease and death.

The term "non-essential" may be misleading. Although histidine was once considered an essential amino acid for infants only, subsequent research has determined that histidine may also be essential for adults. Arginine, ornithine, cysteine, cystine, taurine and tyrosine are classified as non-essential amino acids but may be essential for individuals with certain diseases or nutritional concerns. A suboptimal intake of the essential amino acids increases the body's need for the non-essential amino acids.

AMINO ACIDS

ESSENTIAL AMINO ACIDS

These cannot be made in the body and one must consume them in the form of food. They are called essential amino acids. They include:

Threonine, Isoleucine, Leucine, Valine, Phenylalanine, Tryptophan, Methionine and Lysine

The next three are in fact nonessential amino acids but made in inadequate amount in the body, often requires supplementation, so these two are considered in the category of essential amino acids.

Cysteine (Cystine), Histidine and Arginine,

NONESSENTIAL AMINO ACIDS

The following amino acids are synthesized in the body as the body needs them. They are called nonessential amino acids.

Alanine, Glycine, Serine, Tyrosine, Proline, Aspartic acid, Asparagine, Glutamic acid, Glutamine, hydroxyproline, hydroxylysine, ornithine, and Taurine

The following are also considered as amino acid due to their function:

Asparagine, Glutamine, Hydroxyproline and Hydroxylysine

COFACTORS

Compounds used in our body in metabolic conversion processes are known as cofactors. Vitamins and minerals are main cofactors. Some amino acids, fatty acids, and lipoic acids are also considered as cofactors.

COENZYMES

Enzymes need supporting coenzymes for normal function in the cell. These coenzymes are derived from essential nutrients either from vitamins or trace minerals. Enzymes must be bound to their appropriate coenzyme and at an adequate concentration to function efficiently.

FIBERS

Fibers should be part of a healthy diet. There are certain types of fiber that can affect the amount of calcium the body absorbs. Rhubarb, spinach, chard, and beet greens contain oxalate, which may decrease the absorption of calcium. Phytic acid, found in wheat bran, combines with calcium and also decreases its absorption. Fiber, however, is very helpful to the digestive tract, so it is important to balance the level of calcium intake with the amount and type of fiber in the diet. A diet containing up to 35 grams of fiber per day should be adequate for healthy bowel movements, without adversely affecting calcium absorption.

MINERALS

The minerals used in cofactor composition also have a dual nature in that they can be stored in tissue and thus can pose potential toxicity. The minerals are used in innumerable cellular reactions. For example, magnesium is used in over 300 enzyme reactions and zinc is used as a component of over 5,000 reactions in every cell every second of our lives. Copper, iron, cobalt, and others similarly have important roles in healthy metabolic operations.

Nutritional surveys consistently report that most people do not consume adequate amounts of most vitamins and minerals.

FATTY ACIDS

These are the components of dietary fats in the body. They serve as sources of energy, structural components for nerves and cell membranes and as precursors to special class of hormones. Because fatty acids function relative to each other, a balanced intake is crucial for good health. High levels of arachidonic acid relative to GLA or EPA will lead to predominance of inflammatory chemicals in the body which can promote a greater tendency for heart and other inflammatory diseases. Dietary intake of EPA helps balance that. Fish oils have shown to be beneficial because of this reason.

METABOLISM

Metabolism is an extremely complex subject in human biochemistry. There are many metabolic pathways containing thousands of components and reactions. All of them are important to optimal physical, physiological and mental function.

LECITHIN

Every living cell in the human body needs lecithin. Cell membranes, which regulate which nutrients may leave or enter the cell, are largely composed of lecithin. Cell membranes would harden without lecithin. Its structure protects the cells from damage by oxidation. The protective sheaths surrounding the brain are composed of lecithin, and the muscles and nerve cells also contain this essential fatty substance. Lecithin is composed of choline, inositol, and linoleic acids. It acts as an emulsifying agent. Lecithin is considered a "brain food." It is very essential in autistic child's (person's) diet. In an autistic brain, there are less active axons and dendrites (nerve energy transportation). So messages get lost or distorted. The emulsification action of lecithin can make the nerves smooth and open up the transportation channels to allow the messages to be transported.

It helps prevent arteriosclerosis, protects against cardiovascular disease, increases brain function, and promotes energy. It promotes better digestion of fats and helps disperse cholesterol in water and removes it from the body. The vital organs and arteries are protected from fatty build-up with the inclusion of lecithin in the diet.

Food sources: soybean, eggs, brewer's yeast, grains, legumes, fish, and wheat germ.

The body needs all of the essential vitamins and minerals in proper proportion for its normal function. If there is any deficiency of the vitamins, minerals, trace minerals, or amino acids, it can manifest as some functional disorder or other problem. If it can be found in time and treated or supplemented with appropriate amounts, many unnecessary discomforts can be avoided.

FOOD AND NERVOUS SYSTEM

Autistic people have sluggish liver and spleen function, which leads to poor energy circulation in those areas. Foods with warming properties (more alkaline food) should be eaten more often to improve the energy flow to liver and spleen meridians and organs.

ALKALINE FOODS:

♦ Reduces inflammation.

♦ Helps eliminate brain fog, to think and comprehend faster.

♦ Help to maintain normal blood and nerve circulation.

♦ Help to maintain even distribution of energy throughout the body, Helps reduce the allergic reactions.

♦ Help to maintain overall calmness.

♦ People with alkaline body heal faster and tend to be less emotional.

ACIDIC FOODS:

♦ Cause more inflammation.

♦ Cause more muscle aches and generalized pains and joint pains.

♦ Cause body and brain fatigue.

♦ people with acidic body are slow thinkers, and will have sluggish brain function.

♦ Cause Indigestion, poor assimilation and poor elimination.

♦ Cause poor circulation of blood, lymph and nerve energy.

♦ Wounds heal slowly in acidic body.

♦ Eat more of Alkaline foods and less of Acidic foods.

♦ People with highly acidic body are very emotional.

Alkaline and Acid food groups are given below. Try to eat more alkaline and less acidic foods   Please make sure your child is not allergic to these foods. If you find your child allergic to these foods, please take your child to an NAET practitioner to get him/her treated for the allergy to the item before feeding him/her.

Eggs are alkaline by nature.

Eggs Alkaline: Quail egg, duck egg.

Eggs Mildly Acidic: Chicken egg.

Human milk is alkaline.

Dairy Less Acidic: Aged Cheese, Butter, Cow Milk, Cream, Goat Cheese, Goat Milk, Soy Cheese, and Yogurt.

Dairy More Acidic: Cottage Cheese, Casein, Ice Cream, Milk protein, New Cheese, and Processed Cheese.

Vegetables-alkaline: Arugula, Asparagus, Beet, Bell Pepper, Broccoli, Broccoflower, Brussels Sprout, Burdock, Cabbage, Cauliflower, Celery, Chives, Cilantro, Collard Greens, Cucumber, Daikon, Egg Plant, Endives, Garlic, Ginger Root, Jicama, Kale, Kohlrabi, Lettuce, Lotus Root, Mung Bean, Mushroom, Mustard Greens, Onion, Parsley, Parsnip, Potato, Radish, Rutabaga, Scalion, Seaweed And Other Sea Vegetables, Squash, Sweet Potato, Taro Root, Turmeric, Turnip, And Yam.

Vegetables- Acidic: Carrot, Chard, Lima Bean, Navy Bean, Peanut, Rhubarb, Snow Pea, Spinach, and Zucchini.

Fruits-alkaline: apple, apricot, avocado, banana, blackberry, blueberry, boysenberry, cantaloupe, cherry, citrus, grape, grapefruit, honeydew, lemon, lime, loganberry, mango, nectarine, olive, orange, papaya, peach, pear, persimmon, pineapple, raspberry, raw tomato, strawberry, tangerine, and watermelon.

Fruits-acidic: Canned Fruit, Cherimoya, Cooked Tomato, Cranberry, Date, Dry Fruit, Fig, Guava, Plum, Pomegranate and Prune.

Grains are acidic by nature but some are less acidic and some are more acidic. Try to eat less acidic grains.

Grains - Less Acidic: Amaranth, B vitamins, Brown Rice, Buck Wheat, Farina, Kamut, Kasha, Millet, Oat, Quinoa, Ragi, Sago, Semolina, Spelt, Wheat, White Rice, Wild Rice. Sago grains (produced from sago palm) is a natural tranquilizer. Try to feed them at night to induce good sleep.

Grains - More Acidic: All Purpose Flour, Barley, Bleached Flour, Corn, Rye, Maize, And Oat Bran.

Meat is acidic by nature.

Meat - Less Acidic: Boar, Chicken Egg, Elk, Fish, Game, Gelatin, Goose, Lamb, Mollusks, Organ Meat, Shellfish, Turkey, Venison and wild duck.

Meat-More Acidic: Bear Meat, Beef, Chicken, Lobster, Mussel, Pheasant, Pork, Squid, and Veal.

Dried Bean-Alkaline: Lentils and mung beans

Dried Beans - Acidic: Azuki Beans, Black Eyed Peas, Fava Beans, Green Pea, Kidney Bean, Navy Bean, Pinto Bean, Chick Pea, Garbanzo Bean, Beans, Green Mung Beans, Lentils, Lima Bean, Split Pea, String Bean, White Bean, Red Bean, and Soybean.

Fats -Alkaline: Avocado Oil, Borage Oil, Clarified Butter, Coconut Oil, Cod Liver Oil, Evening Primrose Oil, Flax Seed Oil, Hydrogenated Oil, Linseed Oil, and Olive Oil.

Fats - Less -Acidic: almond oil, canola oil, grapeseed oil, pumpkin seed oil, safflower oil, sesame oil, and sunflower oil.

Fats - More Acidic: Brazil Nut Oil, Chestnut Oil, Cottonseed Oil, Palm Oil, Soy Oil, and Superheated Vegetable Oils.

Nuts- Alkaline: Almond, Cashew, Chestnut, Poppy Seed, Pumpkin Seed, Sesame Seed.

Nuts-Acidic: Brazil Nut, Hazelnut, Peanut, Pecan, Pine Nut, Soy.

Drinks-alkaline: Apple cider vinegar, Cow Milk, Goat Milk, Herbal tea, Honey, Human milk, Maple syrup, Mineral water, Molasses, Rice milk, Rice Syrup, Sugar Cane juice, and Yogurt.

Drinks - acidic: Alcohol, Beer, Cane Sugar, Carbonated Drinks, Chocolate Drinks, Cocoa, Coffee, Cranberry Juice, Ice Cream, Malt, Rice Drink, Rice Milk, Rice Vinegar, Soy Milk, Table salt, White Sugar, White Vinegar, and Yeast,

Juices and drinks: Vegetable juices and broths are preferred to fruit juices. Fruit juices should be taken in minimum quantity (four to six ounces daily). Eating many fruits, and sugar products, drinking a lot of fruit juices etc., can encourage candida growth. Autistic people are susceptible for candida-yeast overgrowth. After NAET, it is okay to have them in moderation. Herbal tea can be used as needed. Avoid carbonated drinks. Instead drink 5-6 glasses of purified or boiled cooled water daily.

Avoid artificial sweeteners, food colorings and additives as much as possible even after NAET treatments. Try to eat more organic, less chemically contaminated, less refined foods. Drink nonallergic water.

12

ERADICATE AUTISM THROUGH NAET

A utistic symptoms in children can manifest in many ways, ranging from mild to moderate to severe, making diagnosis, treatment, and living very difficult. There are no "set" or "typical" behaviors in children with autism. You will hear a variety of terms used to describe different children such as high or low functioning, more or less-abled, autistic-like or autistic tendencies depending upon where the children fall on the continuum. Terms change over the years, but the important thing to remember is that all children are different and their reactions, progress, and length of time necessary to learn proper behaviors, etc. will be different. But they can learn and be productive. It takes time, patience, fortitude, and love.

Children can suffer from various degrees of autism. Their ability to interact with the world will be affected depending on the degree of involvement. No one has definite answers to the cause of autism. From my experience, I believe that allergies play a great role. In the previous chapters we have tried to show the reader how foods, chemicals, drugs, supplements, environmental substances, and emotional events can interfere with mind and body functions and diseases; and they became normal after a series of NAET treatments.

I have treated over a two hundred cases of autism spectrum disorders in my office alone. Close to 90 percent of these children are back in regular schools, leading normal lives. We just completed a case control study on 60 noncommunicative, nonverbalized autistic children - 30 in treatment group and 30 in control group. We began treatments on the treatment group in November 2004. Study just completed this month. Each subject was treated for 50 NAET Allergens. All subjects showed significant improvements in verbal and nonverbal communication skills. 88 percent of these children are attending regular school now. Others need more work before getting their autism labels removed. Control group had no change from last year even though they continued their regular therapies all along. We had promised the control subjects free 50 NAET treatments as we had given to the treatment group once the study was over. They began their NAET treatments this month. The parents of the children are very surprised and amazed at the progress their children made in such a short time. While we were doing the final evaluations, one of the mothers told me that she never ever thought she was going to celebrate another Christmas in her life. Since her only son became so sick she had given up celebrating Christmas. This year she said she is going to make up for the last few years. Tears were rolling down her cheeks while she was telling me this.

Many out of the 8,000 medical practitioners I have trained have shared with me similar satisfactory results with their autistic patients. So far no other treatments have produced such outstanding results in such a short period of time as NAET. As I mentioned earlier, autism is on the rise at an alarming rate. We have to stop this now before it gets out of hand, before many of our children become handicapped, before we lose our children, the productive future citizens of the country–to autism! We need to nip autism in the bud. When we looked at the history of our autistic children, almost every one of them suffered from a number of allergic health disorders. Many are born allergic. Later when they are exposed to a strong allergen like an antibiotic, chemical spray, pesticide, vaccination, immunization or a bacterial or viral toxin, their brain is affected. The nervous system does not know how to correct the unexpected energy disturbance brought on by the unannounced entry of the toxin. Toxins have affected various segments of the brain randomly in these sensitive children. Some children suffered from autism spectrum disorders; some suffered from ADD and ADHD; some suffered from learning disabilities; some suffered from dyslexia; some others suffered from other types of deficiencies of brain function. If the toxins affected any other area of the nervous system, those individuals also suffered from other health disorders like indigestion, skin conditions, joint disorders, poor growth or over growth, etc. along with autism. Varied intensities of these conditions in children are due to several factors:

- The percentage of inheritance of allergic tendency.
- The amount of the toxic exposure.
- The health (immune system) of the individual at the time of exposure.

- The amount of tissue damage or the amount of area suffered from the exposure.

If the speech center, communication center, auditory center, vision center of the brain were affected by the toxin, the child lost the power to properly express the function of those centers. Thus the child became unable to communicate properly, to comprehend adequately, to hear or listen, to feel and respond, or to speak appropriately. Since they could not hear, see, understand, and communicate with others, they began to withdraw and hide within themselves. In this way, they became "autistic" to others.

In some children only one or two centers are affected. Such children may show deficiencies in those areas only. Some may be able to speak but not appropriately; some may be able to see but not speak; some may be able to communicate to some degree; some may be able to hear well but not see clearly. The children with different deficiencies and abilities are grouped together as suffering from autism spectrum disorders. The children with certain essential functions not affected are grouped as high-functional autism, also known as Asperger's syndrome.

We can help all these children with different intensities of autism when we identify the toxin and the area that is affected. Using NAET, we can identify the toxin that triggered the chain event in the child even if it happened years before, then eliminate the adverse reaction between the nervous system and the toxin. Releasing the bond between the nervous system and the toxin will enable the toxin to transport out of the body through appropriate elimination pathways. This will allow the affected area of the nervous system to resume its function to supply the brain or body with appropriate nutrients. Slowly the damaged area will receive nourishments and repair to normal status. When the nerve interference in these centers are removed, the expected functions of the organs will return. Thus these children will hear things again; comprehend again; and manifest communication skills like normal people.

We need to understand the problems first. We need to find the root of their problems that brought them to the present state. This can be done by process of elimination. That is what we do in NAET. We find allergens that produce disturbance in the child's energy field and eliminate them one by one following a special order that has worked best for most people. During this systematic process, the major allergen is detected. In some cases there may be more than a few major allergens causing autism in a child. When the major offenders are removed, body and brain begin healing. Then the brain need to be retrained or reeducated about normal living since they may never have had the chance of normal learning. After the allergies are eliminated, behavior modification becomes easier for parents, children and therapists.

NAET is a simple procedure. We need to make all parents and medical practitioners aware of NAET. This can be done through word of mouth, news media and support groups. Let us join forces with all other autism support groups, autism associations, hospitals and private clinics treating autistic children and adults. We need to encourage all medical professionals and parents to learn NAET, and eradicate this "incurable" brain disorder once and for all using allergy elimination with NAET as the tool.

We need to work on the following areas if we want to eradicate autism permanently.

1. Let's bring all the autistic communities and supporters together to "defeat and destroy" autism and educate them about NAET.

2. Let's teach NST (Chapter 6) to test allergies and other side effects of substances to which we expose our children.

3. Let's make NAET available to all presently affected children and adults.

4. Alert all the parents (present and future) about the importance of testing their children for allergies using NST for all drugs, immunizations, possible chemical and environmental toxins, and foods before they expose their children to these items.

5. If the children are found to be allergic to any of these items, please get them treated with NAET before using them. There are thousands of NAET practitioners all over the world (please look at the web site for practitioner location: www.naet.com).

6. Vaccinations and immunizations can be life-savers to some people. You don't want your child to miss the opportunity of the possible benefits from immunizations if they are as good as they sound. But as a parent, as a doctor, as a health care provider, as a teacher, as a pharmacist, as a vaccine maker, you should be aware of the possible allergic reactions and after-effects if the child is allergic to the immunizations. Ninety percent of such autistic children recovered from autism when they successfully completed the NAET treatments for MMR and DPT immunizations. According to their parents, most of these children were fairly normal until they received the booster doses of immunizations. If the health care providers who injected the children with

vaccines were aware of NST and NAET, they could have prevented these children from reacting.

If there is an allergy, it can harm the child in many ways, one of which may be autism. If one just spends five extra minutes to test a child with NST before injecting the child, one could easily prevent most cases of this disaster–Autism! This goes for parents, doctors, nurses, etc.

Autism can be defeated and destroyed if we work together and follow the six steps listed above.

If parents take their autistic children to an NAET practitioner, after they receive a few basic treatments, most children will become manageable. If they complete the full course of treatments the results will be more than satisfactory in the cases with allergies, (that is giving the benefit of the doubt that there may be some cases without allergies. However, so far I haven't come across any case of autism without an allergy involved.)

The earlier you begin NAET, the faster the results. Children treated under the age of ten have achieved faster results than adults treated for autism with NAET.

Even though autism is currently associated with biological or neurological differences in the brain, the lay public still views autistic children and adults as weird, abnormal and/or eccentric. They may be mistreated by their siblings, relatives, classmates, playmates, and other neighborhood children by name calling and teasing, etc. Parents need to educate relatives, friends, and neighbors. Once people understand, especially other children, they would be less likely to make fun of the child or his/her weaknesses. It is everyone's responsibility, the teacher, counselor, principal, coach, as well as the parents to use appropriate medical terminology to explain the child's health problem to other children, so they will not tease or annoy the child. Not only that, if the need arises, other children should be willing and ready to help the child with any of his/her difficult chores. If the child's root problem is not eliminated, an autistic child's future depends on how the family (parents), siblings, teachers, caretakers and friends present him/her to the world. There are many excellent autistic training centers like "The Option Institute" in this country, which take pride in their productive behavior modification programs and help many autistic children to become normal. Parents should enroll their children in such centers to give them an adequate education. After removing the known allergies, it will take less time for such institutions to do their job.

SELF ESTEEM

There are many ways that parents can begin training even the youngest child to be responsible for his/her actions and build self-confidence as well. Everyday life is not only stressful, but also a challenge with an autistic youngster. However, you should have certain expectations in mind for your child. They give you something to look forward to and build responsibility in your child. He/she should learn to contribute to and be part of the family. Mastering simple tasks will make the child feel good about himself/herself, and build a positive self image. You can do this by developing a daily structured routine: washing, brushing teeth and hair dressing, etc. Allow your child to make simple decisions. Would you like to wear the red shirt or the blue one? Do you want the peanut butter or the turkey sandwich? As the child matures, add responsibilities. By learning to choose he/she learns to make decisions. These tasks may seem small at first but they represent stepping stones to accomplish difficult tasks later on. Your child may be reluctant to cooperate at first but do not give up, take it one step at a time. Remember, the goal is to try to foster as much independence as possible.

BEHAVIOR MANAGEMENT

Tantrums, aggression, unpredictability, repetitive behaviors, and uncontrolled outbursts present some of the greatest challenges to parenting an autistic child. The autistic child's brain works very slowly; sometimes messages are crisscrossed in the brain; their comprehension is limited due to the inefficient nervous system. So you need to get to the child's level and explain things very slowly or talk to the child very softly, word by word if necessary, to make the child understand. If you take enough time and explain, they will understand better and you will get faster results.

By the end of the day you may be completely drained but through consistent, positive behavior modification, your child will begin to react appropriately to situations. The key word is consistent. Reward behaviors you want the child to repeat. Praise him/her, smile, encourage or reward. This form of behavior modification helps your child to learn the correct action or response to a situation. It offers an orderly plan of rewards and punishments (verbal reprimands) to strengthen acceptable responses and discourage unacceptable ones. Be careful not to use behavior modification for everything that happens during the day. Begin by picking one or two behaviors you would like to change. Select a reward for your child. It may be difficult to know what to choose, especially if your child is not responsive. It might be something the child likes to eat, or a hug or smile, a game to play, etc. Try to keep a record of the child's progress with a chart. You might place a sticker or a happy face by the behavior that he/she has done correctly.

Sometimes the behavior may require a " time-out." A "time-out" gives your child a chance to calm down. You simply remove your child from the situation and place him/her in a chair or another room for a specific period of time. You can set a timer and when the timer goes off the child can return to the family. Learning to live within parameters is not easy for a child who is autistic but it is an important step to a productive, responsible life.

EARLY INTERVENTION

The first few years of a child's life are most important to his/her development and so it is with an autistic child. There are special educational services available for children with handicaps or who are at risk of developing them from infancy until the age of five. Early intervention is conducted at home and/or at school. An individual learning plan is designed by an early intervention team, made up of school specialists. The program may include play therapy, teaching social skills, speech therapy etc. It also helps parents cope with everyday problems. There is also time for group activities with normal children, which have proven to improve autistic children's skills. As parents you cannot do everything alone. You need support. Early intervention is a legal right and it has been proven to benefit autistic children by enhancing communication, cognitive, social and self-help skills. The staff can work with you to plan goals based on your child's individual needs.

AS A TEACHER OF AN AUTISTIC CHILD

Teachers need special training in handling difficult cases like autism. Parents should visit the school and observe teachers with special education backgrounds. Usually teachers in pre-schools and other small classes are well trained to observe any imbalances in small children. If the teacher notices any symptoms of autism he/she should give special attention to the child to determine if the observation is true. He/she should meet with the child alone to evaluate the mental status and behavioral pattern of the child, then document the child's behavior and inform the parents, school authorities, and the school psychologist about the findings. This person should work individually with the child and help him/her to improve in the identified areas one at a time. The teacher should pay special attention to introduce the child to the rest of the class and to include him/her in all class activities.

A teacher should know his/her students and make learning fun, making the presentation more interesting by using appropriate visual and auditory aids. Autistic children on the road to recovery can do many things like other normal children. If a child cannot focus, understand, or pay enough attention to things being said or demonstrated by the teacher, the child should be placed among children who understand slightly better. The child will watch the other children and try to imitate them and learn from others. High functioning autistic children cannot focus or concentrate on any task for more than a few minutes at a time. Do not force them. They become frustrated and irritable. By alternating and rotating the visual and auditory stimuli every few minutes, the teacher will encourage the child to be attentive and focus so he/she can learn. Try to bring out the best in the children. Avoid focusing on the child's weakness and avoid speaking negatively about the child to others. Children hear everything and keep it in their memory even though the child appears to be deaf, mute and unresponsive to the surrounding stimuli. The teacher should be patient with the child. Care should be taken not to lose your temper or tease him/her in front of other children. The teacher should not impose excessive punishments for minor things, or forget to reward the child after accomplishing small tasks.

We tend to think that the child cannot understand if he cannot talk, or interact. We have numerous examples to share with you that children appearing to be deaf, mute and inactive can hear every word that is said around them and keep them in their memory and recall them later.

Michael was nine-years-old when his parents brought him to our office for treatment. Michael had never spoken a word until then. He was very restless, never looked you in the eyes while talking to him, appeared as if he did not understand anything that happened around him. Nothing significant happened during the first three treatments. The fourth treatment was for B complex vitamins. He reacted to the B complex treatment differently. Soon after the treatment, he went into a crying spell. He began screaming in his loudest voice and started banging his head on the wall. He couldn't explain how he felt. His symptoms were of some discomfort in his body. I took him into the treatment room and repeated NAET on him every five minutes for three more times. By this time he calmed down. Suddenly, he began yawning. Then he was moved into another room and helped to lie down and the mother was asked to sit with him. In less than five minutes, he was fast asleep. After 20 minutes I rechecked him and then his parents carried the sleeping child home.

During his next visit, he walked into the office along with his parents, singing nursery rhymes. He sat in the waiting room of the clinic and repeated all the nursery rhymes taught in school loud and clear, without a mistake or a pause. His parents were surprised to hear him say the words so clearly, for they had taken it for granted that their son was born unable to speak. This clearly demonstrates that these children hear and store things in their memory ready to retrieve if the situation permits. In his case, an allergy to B vitamins caused him to be unresponsive to everything in his surroundings. When the energy blockage was removed, his restrictions released. The nerves supplying energy to the vocal cords were no longer blocked and the words flowed out of his memory bank. He took many more treatments (about 50 treatments) to eliminate all his known allergies. He is a normal young adult now.

NAET TREATMENTS

An autistic child should be tested and treated for all basic allergies as soon as possible. If possible he/she or the parents should be taught how to self-test for allergies. Make a point to test everything before using them. Any item tested as allergic should be avoided until treatment with NAET.

NUTRITION

After treating for the NAET basics, proper care should be taken to maintain a well balanced diet from the non-allergic food groups. Autistic children and adults deplete B complex vitamins and trace minerals very quickly. These vitamins should be replaced appropriately in their daily diets. They should be encouraged to drink plenty of water (4-6 glasses daily).

BRAIN EXERCISE

Various brain balancing exercises and activities are described in Chapter 8. The parents should make a regular habit of implementing some of those exercises every day to help them maintain a stable mind.

PARENT AND SELF AWARENESS

Parents should be trained to pay attention to the presence of any commonly seen autistic-like behaviors in their children. Any new allergen is capable of reproducing the old physical symptoms or creating a new symptom in a sensitive person. If the parent or child is aware of this, the parent or child will not panic and would be able to pay more attention and make a conscious effort to prevent reacting in front of strangers. Self-instruction, where a child is mentally trained to remind himself/herself is an effective form of mental exercise that can help the child to act and react appropriately in social situations, and can also develop organizational skills. It is okay to take an appropriate drug prescribed by a physician in uncontrollable situations. Have your physician prescribe a non-allergic medication for symptomatic relief. (If the child is allergic to the medication, he/she should be treated for the allergy to the medicine with NAET. The child will not have to take the medication regularly after sufficient NAET treatments have been received. But always make it a point to have the prescription medication available for any emergency that occurs without warning.)

AS A PARENT OF AN AUTISTIC CHILD

As a parent, care of the autistic child should begin before anyone else detects your child's abnormality. There are many books written on normal growth and development of children. All parents should begin reading these books when planning to have a child, and read through these educational materials during pregnancy. Watch the child closely when he/she is growing up. Pay attention to emotional and physical needs wisely. It is advisable to take your infant to a NAET practitioner and get his/her allergies tested and treated if needed before they become a problem. NAET can be used as a good preventive measure.

Parents should make enough time to spend with the child from infancy, by touching, cuddling, caressing, talking to them and visiting places and meeting people with them. Parents should tell the child repeatedly how much they love him/her and how important he/she is in their lives. The child should be made to feel worthy from infancy by the action of the parents. If the infant seems to be restless, hyper, suffers from insomnia, repeated crying spells, temper tantrums, test all his foods, drinks, clothes, chemicals, detergents, toys, etc., by NST. If you find an allergy by NST, please find an NAET practitioner near you and get him/her treated immediately. You may also use the mind calming techniques in Chapter 8 from the very beginning. Whenever such uncomfortable symptoms are exhibited, it is due to some irritation in the body. So hold the child and massage the vertex of the head (top of the head) for a few minutes. This reduces the irritability temporarily. If parents learn to pay enough attention to the child's every day changes, the problem can be caught at an early age and treatment can be provided immediately, sparing them from unnecessary anxious moments in the future.

If parents did not discover the abnormalities in infancy, they do not have to feel guilty or less efficient. Whenever the problem is discovered in your child, begin working with these methods immediately and results will happen before you know it.

A diagnosis of autism in a child affects the entire family. Usually most parents go into a denial stage initially. But it shouldn't last too long. An autistic child brings tremendous inconvenience and readjustments in the parents' and other siblings' lives. But they all should learn to cooperate and help the child to grow up into a normal adult. Family members should be very patient with the child. It doesn't mean that parents shouldn't discipline the child. Take extra time to calmly explain all the rules of the family and what is expected if the child can understand and follow through. If you lay out the rules and never ask the child to follow them, or never check to see if s/he has followed them, children, even an autistic child, will lose respect for the parent. Children watch you closely and if they think they can get away with something they will try every possible avenue. So it is for the parents to teach the child the right course of action from the beginning: putting toys away after play, washing hands after play, teaching him/her to appreciate things, to respect other's toys, books; teaching him/her to say 'thank you' and 'please', etc. Spend time with the child at bedtime telling him/her a bedtime story; giving him/her a gentle vertex massage. If there are more children in the family, consider reading bedtime stories as a group. If the child is not capable of understanding your demands and rules, you still need to take time to explain. As I have described to you earlier, the child understands and stores all messages inside the brain. For some reason the child is not able to respond to you appropriately. When the time comes, he will utilize the knowledge.

If there are siblings, make them take part in the autistic child's daily activities, like washing, dressing, feeding, etc. Siblings will feel very important and give them a sense of responsibility in rearing him/her and this will reduce your burden and solve the sibling rivalry problem. As the child grows up, parents should include him/her in everyday chores, like cleaning house, mowing the lawn, making breakfast, lunch and dinner, setting the dining table, etc. This gives them enough training and confidence, making them feel important in the family, which improves self-image. Improving family life with an autistic child takes understanding, patience, effort and love. Love conquers all obstacles in life. All the children (siblings) should be taught to share and care, love, and support each other from the beginning. With everyone's support and effort, an autistic child should grow up as loved as any other child in a loving, caring atmosphere.

SEEKING PROFESSIONAL HELP

When behavior management enforced by parents and teachers turns ineffective, professional help from counselors and psychotherapists may be necessary to guide an autistic person properly. There are psychologists and therapists with special training and experience in specific areas of behavioral problems of children with different disorders. Their services often prove invaluable in controlling your child. Parents also could benefit from some counseling to cope with the situation.

MEDICATION

Stimulants, antidepressants, beta-blockers, lithium, Naltrexone, and megavitamin therapy have all been used as interventions with autism. However, no single drug or pill has been found to successfully treat the disorder. More research is needed in this area. There are various reasons for someone to depend on medication. Some parents feel they have to keep their children medicated. In some severe cases, it may be necessary to keep them medicated to help them go through school and other activities of life. In some cases, when both parents are working to find enough income to make ends meet, it may be very straining for parents to find the extra time to spend with the child. So keeping the child on medication reduces stress and gets the work done. Some special schools make it mandatory for children to be on medication. Otherwise, it is hard to manage them. Whatever the reason may be to give medication to your child, at least make sure that he/she is not allergic to it. Medication may be okay for a short term. Long term medication should be avoided, if possible. If the child gets allergies eliminated through NAET, he/she may not require long term medication.

AUTISTIC ADULTS

Society today recognizes that everyone, no matter how disabled or handicapped can contribute to the community as a productive citizen. Locating employment to fit your child's needs and abilities may take time and planning, but it is worth it. There are many supportive businesses today that are flexible and open to helping adults with special needs find employment. There are many federal and state agencies that help locate appropriate jobs as well as universities and vocational schools. Some lucky adults get a break and discover NAET. Others will never hear about NAET or will refuse to seek help.

EVALUATING AUTISTIC ADULTS

The procedure for evaluating and establishing the diagnosis for autistic adults is the same as evaluating a child with autism. The classical signs of poor communication skills, lack of social interaction, and sensory impairment are seen in autistic adults just as they are seen in children with this disorder. The impact of autism on an adult might be the same as it is for children. But it is reflected on an adult differently due to the fact that an adult's life is totally different with different demands and expectations. A child is under the care or supervision of a parent, guardian, teacher or care taker. An adult is expected to work, meet other demands of life, live in a community doing some community work, and meet social obligations within the community, family or friends. The impact of life can be overwhelming to an autistic adult.

Autistic adults find it difficult to sit still for a long time anywhere. So they tend to be very restless most of the time. If they could be placed in jobs of their interest, they could work long hours without getting tired. The interest factor should be kept in mind when job placement is arranged.

Autistic adults have difficulty with conversations. They tend to use a limited range of words in their conversations. Sometimes they reverse pronouns using "you" instead of "I." They include irrelevant details, shift topics or persevere on certain topics. They often can recall dates, ages, telephone numbers and addresses as well as factual information like events and measurements. They interrupt people during conversations, get into arguments without respecting others' ideas, and can talk inappropriately or make foolish remarks. Laughing might occur when they are anxious, or crying for no apparent reason. They are unable to understand that other people have beliefs and feelings that might be different from their own. Their interpersonal difficulties create problems in making and keeping friends.

Rote memory is strong in autistic adults (memorizing facts, dates, addresses, etc.), but other types of memory are impaired. Their language difficulties compound their memory deficits.

Organizing materials at work or home is also a problem for autistic adults. They might fall in the group of procrastinators, always late getting up, late getting to work, have difficulty keeping on a time schedule, get anxiety attacks, crying spells, etc.

Some of the above symptoms may be familiar to chemically sensitive people. You don't have to be autistic to experience these symptoms. They are reactions to certain irritations in the body, which could be caused by allergies.

The symptoms of autism vary from person to person and range from mild, to moderate, to severe. Adults with mild symptoms can function and lead a life as close to normal as possible. Others face difficulties in varying degrees.

NAET is not just for autistic children, it can help an autistic person regardless of age or intensity of the problem.

Autism is treatable! Much of what is considered "autism" is caused by allergy. NAET (Nambudripad's Allergy Elimination Technique) has been overwhelmingly successful in treating allergies that have led to autistic-like symptoms. Now that you have read this book, you or your child or loved ones can have a far more promising future than previously thought possible.

WELCOME TO NAET!!!

Say Good-bye to Allergy-related Autism

GLOSSARY

Acetaldehyde: An aldehyde found in cigarette smoke, vehicle exhaust, and smog. It is a metabolic product of Candida albicans and is synthesized from alcohol in the Liver.

Acetylcholine: A neurotransmitter manufactured in the brain, used for memory and control of sensory input and muscular output signals.

Acid: Any compound capable of releasing a hydrogen ion; it will have a pH of less than 7.

Acute: Extremely sharp or severe, as in pain; can also refer to an illness or reaction that is sudden and intense.

Adaptation: Ability of an organism to integrate new elements into its environment.

Addiction: A dependent state characterized by cravings for a particular substance if that substance is withdrawn.

Additive: A substance added in small amounts to foods to alter the food in some way.

Adrenaline: Trademark for preparations of epinephrine, which is a hormone secreted by the adrenal gland. It is used sublingually and by injection to stop allergic reactions.

Aldehyde: A class of organic compounds obtained by oxidation of alcohol. Formaldehyde and acetaldehyde are members of this class of compounds.

Alkaline: Basic, or any substance that accepts a hydrogen ion; its pH will be greater than 7.

Allergenic: Causing or producing an allergic reaction.

Allergen: Any organic or inorganic substance from one's surroundings or from within the body itself that causes an allergic response in an individual is called an allergen. An allergen can cause an IgE antibody mediated or non-IgE mediated response in a person. Some of the commonly known allergens are: pollens, molds, animal dander, food and drinks, chemicals of different kind like the ones found in the food, water, air, fabrics, cleaning agents, environmental materials, detergent, make-up products etc., body secretions, bacteria, virus, synthetic materials, fumes, and air pollution. Emotional unpleasant thoughts like anger, frustration, etc. can also become allergens and cause allergic reactions in people.

Allergic reaction: Adverse, varied symptoms, unique to each person, resulting from the body's response to exposure to allergens.

Allergy: Attacks by the immune system on harmless or even useful things entering the body. Abnormal responses to substances usually well tolerated by most people.

Amino acid: An organic acid that contains an amino (ammonia-like NH_3) chemical group; the building blocks that make up all proteins.

Anaphylactic shock: Also known as anaphylaxis. Usually it happens suddenly when exposed to a highly allergic item. But sometimes, it can also happen as a cumulative reaction. (first two doses of penicillin may not trigger a severe reaction, but the third or fourth could produce an anaphylaxis in some people). An anaphylaxis (this life threatening allergic reaction) is characterized by: an immediate allergic reaction that can cause difficulty in breathing, light headedness, fainting, sensation of chills, internal cold, severe heart palpitation or irregular heart beats, pallor, eyes rolling, poor mental clarity, tremors, internal shaking, extreme fear, angio neurotic edema, throat swelling, drop in blood pressure, nausea, vomiting, diarrhea, swelling anywhere in the body, redness and hives, fever, delirium, unresponsiveness, or sometimes even death.

Antibody: A protein molecule produced in the body by lymphocytes in response to a perceived harmful foreign or abnormal substance (another protein) as a defense mechanism to protect the body. Antibodies protect the body from disease by binding to these organisms and destroying them.

Antigen: Any substance recognized by the immune system that causes the body to produce antibodies; also refers to a concentrated solution of an allergen.

Antihistamine: A chemical that blocks the reaction of histamine that is released by the mast cells and basophils during an allergic reaction. Any substance that slows oxidation, prevents damage from free radicals and results in oxygen sparing.

Arthritis: A medical condition characterized by inflammation of the joints which results in pain and difficulty moving.

Assimilate: To incorporate into a system of the body; to transform nutrients into living tissue.

Asthma: A chronic medical condition where the bronchial tubes (in the lungs) become easily irritated. This leads to constriction of the airways resulting in wheezing, coughing, difficulty breathing and production of thick mucus. The cause of asthma is not yet known but environmental triggers, drugs, food allergies, exercise, infection and stress have all been implicated.

Autism: A chronic developmental disorder usually diagnosed between 18 and 30 months of age. Symptoms include problems with social interaction and communication as well as repetitive interests and activities. At this time, the cause of autism is not known although many experts believe it to be a genetically based disorder that occurs before birth.

Autoimmune: A condition resulting when the body makes antibodies against its own tissues or fluid. The immune system attacks the body it inhabits, which causes damage or alteration of cell function.

Bacteria: Tiny one-celled organisms present throughout the environment that require a microscope to be seen. While not all bacteria are harmful, some cause disease. Examples of bacterial disease include diphtheria, pertussis, tetanus, Haemophilus influenza and pneumococcus (pneumonia).

B cells: Small white blood cells that help the body defend itself against infection. These cells are produced in bone marrow and develop into plasma cells which produce antibodies. Also known as B lymphocytes.

Binder: A substance added to tablets to help hold them together.

Blood brain barrier: A cellular barrier that prevents certain chemicals from passing from the blood to the brain.

Booster shots: Additional doses of a vaccine needed periodically to "boost" the immune system. For example, the tetanus and diphtheria (Td) vaccine which is recommended for adults every ten years.

Buffer: A substance that minimizes changes in pH (Acidity or alkanity).

Candida albicans: A genus of yeast like fungi normally found in the body. It can multiply and cause infections, allergic reactions or toxicity.

Candidiasis: An overgrowth of Candida organisms, which are part of the normal flora of the mouth, skin, intestines and vagina.

Carbohydrate, complex: A large molecule consisting of simple sugars linked together, found in whole grains, vegetables, and fruits. This metabolizes more slowly into glucose than refined carbohydrate.

Carbohydrate, refined: A molecule of sugar that metabolizes quickly to glucose. Refined white sugar, white rice, white flour are some of the examples.

Catalyst: A chemical that speeds up a chemical reaction without being consumed or permanently affected in the process.

Cerebral allergy: Mental dysfunction caused by sensitivity to foods, chemicals, environmental substances, or other substances like work materials etc.

Chronic: Of long duration.

Chronic fatigue syndrome: A syndrome of multiple symptoms most commonly associated with fatigue and reduced energy or no energy.

Crohn's disease: An intestinal disorder associated with irritable bowel syndrome, inflammation of the bowels and colitis.

Cumulative reaction: A type of reaction caused by an accumulation of allergens in the body.

Cytokine Immune system's second line of defense. Examples of cytokines are interleukin 2 and gamma interferon.

Desensitization: The process of building up body tolerance to allergens by the use of extracts of the allergenic substance.

Detoxification: A variety of methods used to reduce toxic materials accumulated in body tissues.

Digestive tract: Includes the salivary glands, mouth, esophagus, stomach, small intestine, portions of the liver, pancreas, and large intestine.

Disorder: A disturbance of regular or normal functions.

Dust: Dust particles from various sources irritate sensitive individual causing different respiratory problems like asthma, bronchitis, hay-fever like symptoms, sinusitis, and cough.

Dust mites: Microscopic insects that live in dusty areas, pillows, blankets, bedding, carpets, upholstered furniture, drapes, corners of the houses where people neglect to clean regularly.

Eczema: An inflammatory process of the skin resulting from skin allergies causing dry, itchy, crusty, scaly, weepy, blisters or eruptions on the skin. Skin rash frequently caused by allergy.

Edema: Excess fluid accumulation in tissue spaces. It could be localized or generalized.

Electromagnetic: Refers to emissions and interactions of both electric and magnetic components. Magnetism arising from electric charge in motion. This has a definite amount of energy.

Elimination diet: A diet in which common allergenic foods and those suspected of causing allergic symptoms have been temporarily eliminated.

Endocrine: refers to ductless glands that manufacture and secrete hormones into the blood stream or extracellular fluids.

Endocrine system: Thyroid, parathyroid, pituitary, hypo-thalamus, adrenal glands, pineal gland, gonads, the intestinal tract, kidneys, liver, and placenta.

Endogenous: Originating from or due to internal causes.

Environment: A total of circumstances and/or surroundings in which an organism exists. May be a combination of internal or external influences that can affect an individual.

Environmental illness: A complex set of symptoms caused by adverse reactions of the body to external and internal environments.

Enzyme: A substance, usually protein in nature and formed in living cells, which starts or stops biochemical reactions.

Eosinophil: A type of white blood cell. Eosinophil levels may be high in some cases of allergy or parasitic infestation.

Exogenous: Originating from or due to external causes.

Extract: Treatment dilution of an antigen used in immunotherapy, such as food, chemical, or pollen extract.

Fibromyalgia: An immune complex disorder causing general body aches, muscle aches, and general fatigue.

"Fight" or "flight": The activation of the sympathetic branch of the autonomic nervous system, preparing the body to meet a threat or challenge.

Food addiction: A person becomes dependent on a particular allergenic food and must keep eating it regularly in order to prevent withdrawal symptoms.

Food grouping: A grouping of foods according to their botanical or biological characteristics.

Free radical: A substance with unpaired electrode, which is attracted to cell membranes and enzymes where it binds and causes damage.

Gastrointestinal: Relating both to stomach and intestines.

Heparin: A substance released during allergic reaction. Heparin has antiinflammatory action in the body.

Histamine: A body substance released by mast cells and basophils during allergic reactions, which precipitates allergic symptoms.

Holistic: Refers to the idea that health and wellness depend on a balance between physical (structural) aspects, physiological (chemical, nutritional, functional) aspects, emotional and spiritual aspects of a person.

Homeopathic: Refers to giving minute amounts of remedies that in massive doses would produce effects similar to the condition being treated.

Homeostasis: A state of perfect balance in the organism also called "Yin-yang" balance. The balance of functions and chemical composition within an organism that results from the actions of regulatory systems.

Hormone: A chemical substance that is produced in the body, secreted into body fluids, and is transported to other organs, where it produces a specific effect on metabolism.

Hydrocarbon: A chemical compound that contains only hydrogen and carbon.

Hypersensitivity: An acquired reactivity to an antigen that can result in bodily damage upon subsequent exposure to that particular antigen.

Hyperthyroidism: A condition resulting from over-function of the thyroid gland.

Hypoallergenic: Refers to products formulated to contain the minimum possible allergens and some people with few allergies can tolerate them well. Severely allergic people can still react to these items.

Hypothyroidism: A condition resulting from under-function of the thyroid gland.

IgA: Immunoglobulin A, an antibody found in secretions associated with mucous membranes.

IgD: Immunoglobulin D, an antibody found on the surface of B-cells.

IgE: Immunoglobulin E, an antibody responsible for immediate hypersensitivity and skin reactions.

IgG: Immunoglobulin G, also known as gammaglobulin, the major antibody in the blood that protects against bacteria and viruses.

IgM: Immunoglobulin M, the first antibody to appear during an immune response.

Immune system: The body's defense system, composed of specialized cells, organs, and body fluids. It has the ability to locate, neutralize, metabolize and eliminate unwanted or foreign substances.

Immunocompromised: A person whose immune system has been damaged or stressed and is not functioning properly.

Immunity: Inherited, acquired, or induced state of being, able to resist a particular antigen by producing antibodies to counteract it. A unique mechanism of the organism to protect and maintain its body against adversity by its surroundings.

Inflammation: The reaction of tissues to injury from trauma, infection, or irritating substances. Affected tissue can be hot, reddened, swollen, and tender.

Inhalant: Any airborne substance small enough to be inhaled into the lungs; eg., pollen, dust, mold, animal danders, perfume, smoke, and smell from chemical compounds.

Intolerance: Inability of an organism to utilize a substance.

Intracellular: Situated within a cell or cells.

Intradermal: method of testing in which a measured amount of antigen is injected between the top layers of the skin.

Ion: An atom that has lost or gained an electron and thus carries an electric charge.

Kinesiology: Science of movement of the muscles.

Latent: Concealed or inactive.

Leukocytes: White blood cells.

Lipids: Fats and oils that are insoluble in water. Oils are liquids in room temperature and fats are solid.

Lymph: A clear, watery, alkaline body fluid found in the lymph vessels and tissue spaces. Contains mostly white blood cells.

Lymphocyte: A type of white blood cell, usually classified as T-or B-cells.

Macrophage: A white blood cell that kills and ingests microorganisms and other body cells.

Masking: Suppression of symptoms due to frequent exposure to a substance to which a person is sensitive.

Mast cells: Large cells containing histamine, found in mucous membranes and skin cells. The histamine in these cells are released during certain allergic reactions.

Mediated: Serving as the vehicle to bring about a phenomenon, eg., an IgE-mediated reaction is one in which IgE changes cause the symptoms and the reaction to proceed.

Membrane: A thin sheet or layer of pliable tissue that lines a cavity, connects two structures, selective barrier.

Metabolism: Complex chemical and electrical processes in living cells by which energy is produced and life is maintained. New material is assimilated for growth, repair, and replacement of tissues. Waste products are excreted.

Migraine: A condition marked by recurrent severe headaches often on one side of the head, often accompanied by nausea, vomiting, and light aura. These headaches are frequently attributed to food allergy.

Mineral: An inorganic substance. The major minerals in the body are calcium, phosphorus, potassium, sulfur, sodium, chloride, and magnesium.

Mucous membranes: Moist tissues forming the lining of body cavities that have an external opening, such as the respiratory, digestive, and urinary tracts.

Muscle Response Testing (MRT) or Neuromuscular Sensitivity Testing (NST): A testing technique based on kinesiology to test allergies by comparing the strength of a muscle or a group of muscles in the presence and absence of the allergen.

NAET: (Nambudripad's Allergy Elimination Techniques): A technique to eliminate allergies permanently from the body towards the treated allergen. Developed by Dr. Devi S. Nambudripad and practiced by more than 8,000 medical practitioners worldwide. This technique is natural, non-invasive, and drug-free. It has been effectively used in treating all types of allergies and problems arising from allergies. It is taught by Dr. Nambudripad in Buena Park, CA. to currently licensed medical practitioners. If you are interested in learning more about NAET, or NAET seminars, please visit the website: www.naet.com.

Nervous system: A network made up of nerve cells, the brain, and the spinal cord, which regulates and coordinates body activities.

NTP: A series of standard diagnostic tests used by NAET practitioners to detect allergies is called "Nambudripad's Testing Procedures"or NTP.

Neurotransmitter: A molecule that transmits electrical and/or chemical messages from nerve cell (neuron) to nerve cell.

Nutrients: Vitamins, minerals, amino acids, fatty acids, and sugar (glucose), which are the raw materials needed by the body to provide energy, effect repairs, and maintain functions.

Organic foods: Foods grown in soil free of chemical fertilizers, and without pesticides, fungicides and herbicides.

Outgasing: The releasing of volatile chemicals that evaporate slowly and constantly from seemingly stable materials such as plastics, synthetic fibers, or building materials.

Overload: The overpowering of the immune system due to massive concurrent exposure or to low level continuous exposure caused by many stresses, including allergens.

Parasite: An organism that depends on another organism (host) for food and shelter, contributing nothing to the survival of the host.

Pathogenic: Capable of causing disease.

Pathology: The scientific study of disease; its cause, processes, structural or functional changes, developments and consequences.

Pathway: The metabolic route used by body systems to facilitate biochemical functions.

Peakflow meter: An inexpensive, valuable tool used in measuring the speed of the air forced out of the lungs and helps to monitor breathing disorders like asthma.

Petrochemical: A chemical derived from petroleum or natural gas.

pH: A scale from 1 to 14 used to measure acidity and alkanity of solutions. A pH of 1-6 is acidic; a pH of 7 is neutral; a pH of 8-14 is alkaline or basic.

Postnasal drip: The leakage of nasal fluids and mucus down into the back of the throat.

Precursor: Anything that precedes another thing or event, such as physiologically inactive substance that is converted into an active substance that is converted into an active enzyme, vitamin, or hormone.

Prostaglandin: A group of unsaturated, modified fatty acids with regulatory functions.

Radiation: The process of emission, transmission, and absorption of any type of waves or particles of energy, such as light, radio, ultraviolet or X-rays.

Receptor: Special protein structures on cells where hormones, neurotransmitters, and enzymes attach to the cell surface.

Respiratory system: The system that begins with the nostrils and extends through the nose to the back of the throat and into the larynx and lungs.

Rotation diet: A diet in which a particular food and other foods in the same "family" are eaten only once every four to seven days.

Sensitivity: An adaptive state in which a person develops a group of adverse symptoms to the environment, either internal or external. Generally refers to non-IgE reactions.

Serotonin: A constituent of blood platelets and other organs that is released during allergic reactions. It also functions as a neurotransmitter in the body.

Sublingual: Under the tongue, method of testing or treatment in which a measured amount of an antigen or extract is administered under the tongue, behind the teeth. Absorption of the substance is rapid in this way.

Supplement: Nutrient material taken in addition to food in order to satisfy extra demands, effect repair, and prevent degeneration of body systems.

Susceptibility: An alternative term used to describe sensitivity.

Symptoms: A recognizable change in a person's physical or mental state, that is different from normal function, sensation, or appearance and may indicate a disorder or disease.

Syndrome: A group of symptoms or signs that, occurring together, produce a pattern typical of a particular disorder.

Synthetic: Made in a laboratory; not normally produced in nature, or may be a copy of a substance made in nature.

Systemic: Affecting the entire body.

Target organ: The particular organ or system in an individual that will be affected most often by allergic reactions to varying substances.

Toxicity: A poisonous, irritating, or injurious effect resulting when a person ingests or produces a substance in excess of his or her tolerance threshold.

RESOURCES

Nambudripad's Allergy Research Foundation
6714 Beach Blvd., Buena Park, CA 90621
(714) 523-8900 Fax (714) 523-3068
website: www.naet.com
email: naet@earthlink.net

American Association of University
Affiliated Programs for Persons with Developmental Disabilities
8630 Fenton Street, Ste. 410
Silver Spring, MD 20910
(301) 588-8252

Autism Outreach Project
123 Franklin Corner Road, Ste. 215
Lawrenceville, NJ 98648
(609) 895-0190

Autism Research Institute
4182 Adams Avenue
San Diego, CA 92116
(619) 281-7165

Autism Society of America
7910 Woodmont Avenue, Ste. 650
Betthesda, MD 200814
(800) 3-AUTISM

Autism Support Center
64 Holten Street
Danvers, MA 01923
(508) 777-9135

Autism Research Center
1002 East McDowell Road, Suite A
Phoenix, AZ 85006

Center for the Study of Autism
2207 B Portland Road
Newberg, OR 97132
(503) 538-9045

National Information Center for
Children and Youth with Disabilities
P.O. Box 1492
Washington, D.C. 20013
(800) 695-0285

Metagenics
100 Avenida La Plata
San Clemente, CA 92673
(949) 366-0818/ 800-692-9400
Nutritional supplements

Ever Green Herbs (Chinese formula)
1124 N. Hacienda Blvd.
La Puente, CA 91626
(626) 916-1070

Integrative Therapeutics (contact for endfatigue enfusion –the multivitamin-mineral formula)
Jacob Teitelbaum MD
CFS/Fibromyalgia Therapies
Author of the best selling book *"From Fatigued to Fantastic!"* and *"Three Steps to Happiness!*
Healing Through Joy"
"Pain Pain Go away"
(410) 573-5389
www.EndFatigue.com

ORGANIZATIONS

Allergy Induced Autism is a U.K. based charity dedicated to identifying the underlying causes and biochemical effects of autistic spectrum disorders.

Information on Autism Research Institute and on Gluten/Casein Intolerance in Autism - Available on ARI website.

There's a new group for autistic children whose parents are not giving them gluten or casein: The Autism Network for Dietary Intervention (ANDI), begun by Lisa Lewis and Karyn Seroussi.

 The Center for the Study of Autism has many articles on "Allergies and Food Sensitivities", DMG, and articles on intervention.

The Cure Autism Now Foundation is dedicated to finding effective biological treatments, preventaion, and a cure for autism and related disorders.

The National Alliance for Autism Research is families and scientists promoting biomedical research in autism.

The Feingold Diet is "a dietary connection to better behavior, learning, and health." Also see their The Cave Man's Feingold Diet. Requires registration.

 All of the above are available through ARI Website.

BIBLIOGRAPHY

Arbuckle, B.E. Cranial birth injuries. Academy of Applied Osteopathy, yearbook 1945:63.

Arbuckle, B.E. Early cranial considerations. JAOA 48(2):315-320. Arbuckle, B.E. Effects of uterine forceps upon the fetus. JAOA 54(5)#9:499-508.

Asperger, H. (1979). Problems of Infantile Autism. Communication. 13, 45-52.

Autism Autoimmunity Project, "The causes of autism and the need for immunological research: Excerpts from the autism literature," available on the internet at //http/libnt2.lib.tcu.edu/staff/lruede/immresearch.html (Autism Autoimmunity Project, www.gri.net/truegrit) "U.S. Officials investigate 'cluster' of autism in New Jersey Town," CNN, February 1, 1999.

Autism Research Institute.Autism Treatment Evaluation Checklist (ATEC) (Letter to Practitioners and Researchers). Accessed March 20, 2005. Available from: http://www.autismeval.com/ari-atec/research.html

Autism Society of America. Autism Information. Accessed March 13, 2005. Bethesda, MD: Autism Society of America.Available from: http://www.autism-society.org/site/PageServer/ Page name= all about autism &JServSessionIdr001= 47 zepteww1.app2a

Baron, Judy and Sean Barron. There's a Boy in Here. New York: Simon and Shuster, 1993.

Baron-Cohen, Simon, and Patrick Bolton. Autism: The Facts. Oxford: Oxford University Press, 1993.

Bauman, M.L., R.A. Filipek and T.L. Kemper. 1997. Early infantile autism. International review of neurobiology 41:367-386.

Bettelheim, B. The Empty Fortress: Infantile Autism and the Birth of Self. New York: Free Press, 1967.

Betts, Carolyn. A Special Kind of Normal. New York Scribner, 1983.

Bodfish JW. Treating the core features of autism: Are we there yet? *Mental Retardation and Developmental Disabilities Research Review*, 2004;10: 318-326.

Brandl, Cherlene. *Facilitated Communication: Case Studies--* See Us Smart! Ann Arbor Maine: Robbie Dean Press, 1999.

Bristol, M., D.J. Cohen et al. 1996. *State of science of autism:* report to the National Institutes of Health. Journal of autism and developmental disorders 26(2):121-154.

Callahan, Mary. *Fighting for Tony.* New York: Simon and Schuster, 1997.

Capps, L., Sigman, M., and P. Mundy. *Attachment Security in Children with Autism. Development and Psychopathology,* 6, 24999-261.

Castleman, *Michael. Nature's Cures.* Emmaus, PA: Rodale Press, 1996.

Chopra, Deepak. *Perfect Health---The Complete Mind/Body Guide.* New York: Harmony Books, 1991.

Chugani, D., O. Musik et al. 1997. *Altered serotonin synthesis in the dentatothalamococrtical pathway in autistic boys.* Annals of Neurology 42(10)#4:666-669.

Cohen, D.J., Donnellan, A. and R. Paul (eds). *Handbook of Autism and Pervasive Development Disorders.* New York: Wiley, 1987.

Dawson, G., ed. 1989. *Autism: nature, diagnosis and treatment.* New York. Guilford Press 23A. Wales, pers. comm. 1999. My own pers. experience.

Cook, E.H., Jr., 1996. *Brief report: pathophysiology of autism:* neurochemistry. Journal of autism and developmental disorders 26(2):221-225.

Courchesne, E., J. Townsend, et al. 1994. *The brain in infantile autism: posterior fossa structures are abnormal.* Neurology 44:214-223.

Courchesne, E., R. Yeung-Courchesne, et al. 1988. *Hypoplasis of cerebellar lobules VI-VII in infant autism.* New England Journal of Medicine 318:1349-1354.

Courchesne, E. 1999. Correspondence re: *an MRI study of autism: the cerebellum revisited.* Neurology 52:1106.

Diagnostic and Statistical Manual of Mental Disorders. (4th ed.). Washington, D.C: American Psychiatric Association, 1994.

Diagnostic and Statistical Manual of Mental Disorders. DSM IV-TR, *(4th ed.).* Washington, D.C: American Psychiatric Association, 2000.

Di Martino A, Melis G, Cianchetti C, Zuddas A. Methylphenidate for pervasive developmental disorders: safety and efficacy of acute single dose test and ongoing therapy: an open-pilot study. *J Child Adolesc Psychopharmacol.* 2004; 14: 207-18.

DeLong, G.R. 1999. *Autism: new data suggesting new hypothesis:* views and reviews. Neurology 52:911-916.

Doctors warn developmental disabilities epidemic from toxins, LDA (Learning Disabilities Association of America) News briefs 35.4 (July/August 2000): 3; executive summary from the report by the Greater Boston Physicians for Social Responsiblity, In *"Harm's way–Toxic Threats to Child development."*

Available at www.igc.org/psr/ihw.htm;for LDA, www.ldanatl.org.

Dillon, Katleen M. Living with Autism: *The Parents' Stories. Boone*, NC: Parkway, 1995.

Edelson, stephen, Ph.D., Rimland, Bernard, Ph.D. *Treating Autism*, Autism Research Institute, San Diego, 2003

Ernst, M., A.J. Zametkin, et al. 1997. *Low medical prefrontal dopaminergic activity in autistic children.* The Lancet 350(8):638.

Firth, U. *Autism and Asperger Syndrome.* Cambridge, England: University Press, 1991.

Frymann, V.M. *Relation of disturbances of craniosacral mechanisms to symptomalogy of the newborn:* a study of 1,250 infants. JAOA 65(10):1059-1075.

Fryman, V.M., (1976) *Trauma of birth.* Osteopathic Annals 4(22):8-14.

Frymann, V.M., R.E. Carney, et al. *Effect of osteopathic medical management on neurologic development in children.* JAOA 92(6):729-744.

Frymann, V.M. *Learning difficulties of children viewed in the light of osteopathic concept.* JAOA 76(1):46-61.

Garrison, William. Small Bargains: *Children in Crisis and the Meaning of Parental Love.* New York: Simon and Schuster, 1993.

Gerlach, Elizabeth K. *Autism Treatment Guide.* Four-Leaf Press, 1993.

Gillman JT, Tuchman RF. Autism and associated behavioral disorders:

pharmacotherapeutic intervention. *Ann Pharmacother,* 1995;29: 47-56.

Grandin, Temple, and Margaret M. Scariano. *Emergence: Labeled Autistic.* New York: Warner Books, 1996.

Harrington, Kathie. For Parents and Professionals: *Autism. Lingui Systems,* 1998.

Jealous, J.1997. Conservations: *healing and the natural world.* Alternative therapies 3(1):68-75.

Kane, P. 1997. *Peroxisomal Disturbances in Autistic Spectrum Disorder.* Journal of Orthomolecular Medicine 12 (4):207-218.

Kephart, Beth. A Slant of the Sun: *One Child's Courage.* W.W. Norton: 1998.

Kathleen F. Jackson, Autism case Study, Journal Of NAET Energetic And Complementary Medicine, Vol.1, No.1., 2005.

Kaufman, Barry Neil. *Son-Rise.* New York: Harper and Row, 1976.

Kaufman, Barry Neil and Samarhia Lyte Kaufman. *Son-Rise: The Miracle Continues.* Kramer, 1994.

Landrigan, P., and J. Witte. *Neurologic Disorders Following Measles Virus Vaccinations.* JAMA233: 1459 (1973)

Lawrence Lavine, *"Osteopathic and alternative medicine aspects of autistic spectrum disorders,"* article on the internet (available at trainland.tripod.com/lawrencelavine.htm).

Lippincott, R.C. *Cranial Osteopathy.* AAO Year Book 1947:103-111.

Lynne Cannon, *"The Environment and Learning Disabilities,"* LDA Newsbriefs 35:4 (July/August 2000): 1; forLDA, www.ldanatl.org.

Lynne Cannon, *"The Environment and Learning Disabilities,"* LDA Newsbriefs 35:4 (July/August 2000): 1; for LDA, www.ldanatl.org.

Madaule, Paul. When Listening Comes Alive: A Guide to Effective Learning and communication, Norval, Ontario:Moulin, 1994.

Manning, Anita. 1999. *Vaccine-autism link feared. USA Today,* 16 Aug. 99.

Matson, J.L., D.A. Benavidez et al. 1996. *Behavioral treatment of autistic persons:* a review of research from 1980 to the present. Research in developmental disabilities 17(6):433-465.

McBean, Eleanor. *Vaccinations Do Not Protect.* Manachaea, TX: Health

Excellence Systems, 1991.

McGilvery, Robert W., and Gerald W. Goldstein. *Biochemistry---A Functional Approcah.* Phillllladphia, PA: W.B. Saunders Company, 1983.

Miller, Neil Z. Vaccines: *Are They Really Safe and Effective?* Santa Fe, New Mexico: New Atlantian Press, 1992.

Ming X, Julu PO, Wark J, Apartopoulos F, Hansen S. Discordant mental and physical efforts in an autistic patient. *Brain and Development*, 2004; 26: 519-524.

Nambudripad's Allergy Elimination Techniques. What is NAET? Accessed March 2, 2005. Available from: http://www.naet.com/subscribers/index.html

Nambudripad, D. S., *Say Good-bye to Illness,* English, 3rd. Ed., Buena Park, California, Delta Publishing, 2002.

Nambudripad, D. S., *Say Good-bye to Illness,* French Edition, Buena Park, California, Delta Publishing, 2001.

Nambudripad, D. S., *Say Good-bye to Illness,* Spanish Edition, Buena Park, California, Delta Publishing, 1999.

Nambudripad, D. S., *The NAET Guide Book, 6th Edition,* Buena Park, California, Delta Publishing, 2004.

Nambudripad, D. S., *The NAET Guide Book, French Edition,* Buena Park, California, Delta Publishing, 2003.

Nambudripad, D. S., *The NAET Guide Book, German Edition,* Buena Park, California, Delta Publishing, 2004.

Nambudripad, D. S., *Say Good-bye to Allergy-related Autism,* 2nd. Ed., Buena Park, California, Delta Publishing, 2004.

Nambudripad, D. S., *Say Good-bye to ADD and ADHD,* Buena Park, California, Delta Publishing, 1999.

Nambudripad, D. S., *Say Good-bye to Your Allergies,* Buena Park, California, Delta Publishing, 2004.

Nambudripad, D. S., *Say Good-bye to Children's Allergies.,* Buena Park, California, Delta Publishing, 1999.

Nambudripad, D. S., *Living Pain Free.,* A Self-help Book on Acupressure Therapy, Buena Park, California, Delta Publishing, 1997.

Nambudripad, D. S., *Freedom From Environmental Sensitivities,* Buena Park, California, Delta Publishing, 2005.

Nambudripad, D. S., *Say Good-bye to Asthma,* Buena Park, California, Delta Publishing, 2004.

No authors listed. Risperidone in the treatment of disruptive behavioral symptoms in children with autistic and other pervasive developmental disorders. *Child Care Health Dev.* 2005; 31: 247-248.

Oppenheim, Rosalind. *Effective Teaching Methods for Autistic Children.* Springfield, Illinois: Charles C. Thomas, 1974.

Orange County register, *Newsbriefs: Focus/Health,* November 19, 2003

Pangborn, Jon, B. PhD., and Sidney Baker, M.D. *Biomedical Assessment Options For Children With Autism And Related problems*, Autism research Institute, San Diego, 2002.

Piaget, J. *The Construction of Reality in the Child.* New York: W.W. Norton, 1962.

Piven, J., E. Nehme, et al. 1992. *Magnetic resonance imaging in autism: measurement of the cerebellum, pons, and fourth ventricle.* Biologic Psychiatry 31:491-504.

Rutter, M. Autistic Children: *Infancy to Adulthood. Seminars in Psychiatry and Allied Disciplines,* 24, 513-531.

Rapp, Doris. *Is This Your Child?* New York: William Morrow and Company, 1991.

Rapp, Doris. *Our Toxic World: A Wake Up Call. Environmental Medical Research Foundation, Buffalo, NY.. Tel. 1-800-787-8780.* Website: www.drrapp.com

Rapin, I., and R. Katzman, 1998. *Neurobiology of autism.* Annals of neurology 43(1):7-14.

Rapin, I. 1999. *Autism in search of a home in the brain.* Neurology 52:902-904.

Rea, William J. *Chemical Sensitivity.* Boca Raton, FL: Lewis Publishers, 1996.

Rellini E, Tortolani D, Trillo S, Carbone S, Montecchi F. Childhood Autism Rating Scale (CARS) and Autism Behavior Checklist (ABC) Correspondence and Conflicts with DSM-IV Criteria in Diagnosis of Autism. *J Autism Dev Dis.* 2004; 34: 703-708.

Richard Leviton, *"The Healthy Living Space,"* Charlotteville, Virginia: Hampton Roads, 2001:2.

Richard Leviton, *"The Healthy Living Space,"* Charlotteville, Virginia: Hampton Roads, 2001:3.

Rimland, Bernard. *Controversies in the Treatment of Autistic Children: Vitamin and Drug Therapy,* J. Child Neurol. 3 Suppl: S6-16, 1988.

Rimland, Bernard. *Secretin Update.* Autism Research Review International. March, 1999.

Rimland, Bernard. Vaccinations: *The Overlooked Factors. Autism* Research Review International, 1998.

Rimland, Bernard. *Candida-Caused Autism?* Autism Research Review International, 1988.

Rimland, Bernard, Ph.D., in *"Defeat Autism Now (*DAN!) Mercury Detoxification Consensus Group Position Paper,"* Autism research institute, San Diego, California, May 2001:3.

Sanua, VD. *Studies in Infantile Autism.* Child Psychiatry Hum. Dev. 19(3):207-27, 1989.

Smalley, S.L., Asarnow, R.F. and A. Spence. (1988) *Autism and Genetics:* A Decade of Research. Archives of General Psychiatry, 455, 953-961.

Smalley, S.L. and F. Collins. 1996. *Brief report: genetic, prenatal and immunologic factors.* Journal of autism and developmental disorders 26(2):195-198.

Smith, M.D. *Autism and Life in the Community:* Successful Interventions for Behavioral Challenges. Paul Brooks, 1990.

Smith, CW, Electromagnetic Man: *Health and Hazard in the Electrical Environment*, Martin's Press, 1989, 90, 97.

Smith CW, Environmental Medicine: *Electromagnetic Aspects of Biological Cycles,* 1995:9(3):113-118

Smith CW., Electrical Environmental Influences on the Autonomic Nervous System, 11th. Intl. Symp. on *"Man and His Environment in Health and Disease,"* Dallas, Texas, February 25-28, 1993

Smith CW., Electromagnetic Fields and the Endocrine System, 10th. Intl. Symp. on *"Man and His Environment in Health and Disease,"* Dallas, Texas, February 27- March 1, 1992

Smith CW., Basic Bioelectricity: Bioelectricity and Environmental Medicine, 15th. Intl. Symp., on *"Man and His Environment in Health and Disease,"* Dallas, Texas, February 20-23, 1997. (Audio Tapes from:

Professional Audio Recording, 2300 Foothill Blvd. #409, La Verne, CA

Speer, F., ed. 1970. *Allergy of the nervous system.* Springfield: Charles C. Thomas pub.

Sutherland, W.G. Bent Twigs: *compression of the condylar parts of the occiput.* Teachings in the science of osteopathy. Ed. A.L. Wales. Rurda Press, 1990, 107-117.

Sutherland, W.G. (1943) *The Cranial Bowl.* JAOA 48(4):348-53.

Sutherland, A.S., and A.L. Wales, eds. 1967. *Contributions of thought*: collected writings of William Gamer Sutherland 1914-1 954. The Sutherland Cranial Teaching Foundation.

Sutherland, W.G. (1939) *The cranial bowl:* a treatise relating to cranial articular mobility, cranial articular lesions, and cranial technique.Free Press, 1994.

State of California. California Health and Human Services Agency. Dept of Developmental Services. *Changes in the population of persons with Autism/PDD in California's Developmental Services* System:1987 through 1998. A report to the Legislature: March 1, 1999.

Stehl, Annabel. *The Sound of a Miracle, A Child's Triumph Over Autism.* Doubleday, 1991

Stehl, Annabel. Dancing in the Rain: *Stories of Exceptional Progress by Parents of Children with Special Needs* Georgiana, 1995

Strom, Charles M. Heredity and Ability: *How Genetics Affects Your Child and What You Can Do About It* New York: Plenum Press, 1990

Susser, M. 1973. *Causal thinking in the health sciences: concepts and strategies of epidemiology.* 3rd ed. New York: Oxford UP.

Sui, Choa Kok, Pranic Healing, Samuel Wiser, 1990

"The Holistic Physician–Autism," Alternative Medicine Digest 14 (September 1996):20.

Teitlebaum, Jacob, M.D., *From Fatigued to Fantastic*, 1st ed., 1996, 2nd. ed., 2001, Avery Penguin Putnam

Tager-Flusberg, H. *Sentence Comprehension in Autistic Children.* Applied Psycholinguistics, 2, 5-24

The Journal of NAET Energetics and Complementary Medicine, Vol.1, No.1,

Spring 2005.

U.S. Department of Health and Human services, *"Mental health: A report of the Surgeon General,"* Rockville, Maryland: U.S. Department of Health and Human Services, Substance Abuse and Mental H e a l t h Services Administration, Center for Mental health services, National Institute of Health, National Institute of Mental Health, 1999.

Volkmar, F.R. and D.J. Cohen. (1991). *Debate and Argument: The Ultility of the Term Pervasive Developmental Disorder.* Journal of Child Psychology and Psychiatry. 32, 1171-1172

Volkmar, F.R., Paul R., and D. Cohen. (1985). *The Use of "Asperger's Syndrome."* Journal of Autism and Developmental Disorders, 15, 437-439

Wales, A.L. *Cranial diagnosis.* Journal of the Osteopathic Cranial Association 1948:14-23.

Weil, Andrew. *Health and Healing*---Understanding Conventional and Alternative Medicine. Dorling Kindersley, 1995

Wild, Gaynor, and Edward c. Benzel *Essentials of Neurochemistry.* Boston, MA: Joues and Bartlett Publishers, 1994

Williams, Donna. *Nobody Nowhere,* Random House, 1992

Wing, Lorna. *Early Childhood Autism.* Oxford: Pergamon Press, 1976

Wing, Lorna. *Autistic Children:* A Guide for Parents and Professionals, 2nd edition. New York: Brunner/ Mazel, 1985

Weiss, Jordan, M.D., *Psychoenergetics,* 2nd. ed., Oceanview Publishing, 1995

Woods, R.H. 1973. *Structural normalization in infants and children with particular references to disturbances of the central nervous system.* JAOA 72(5):903-08.

Zong, Linda, *Chinese Internal Medicine, lectures* at SAMRA University, Los Angeles, 1985

Case Histories from the Author's private practice,1984-present

Say Good-bye to Allergy-related Autism

Index

Index